HAIR LOSS *in* WOMEN

A catalogue record for this
work is available from the
National Library of Australia

Staveley, Bambi (author)
Hair Loss in Women
ISBN: 978-1-922890-24-5
DEWEY #: 616.546
Self-Help
Health

Typeset Calluna Regular 11.5/19

Written by Bambi Staveley
Book cover design by Bambi Staveley
Book interior design by Green Hill Publishing

HAIR LOSS *in* WOMEN

BAMBI STAVELEY

CONTENTS

Part II: Female pattern hair loss

WHY I WROTE THIS BOOK

Hair loss for a woman can be a devastating blow. A blow to our self-esteem and our very identity.

Like me, you have no doubt been searching the internet for answers, only to discover a world of contradictory information and a sea of so-called magic potions, drops, supplements and miracle cures all competing for our desperate dollar.

You are probably confused by all the conflicting advice, whether from doctors, other women or online charlatans and haircare product companies, all with something to sell. Working your way through this is a daunting task along with the constant worry that you may never get your hair back and living with the fear of going bald.

You may feel like you are carrying this burden alone, but I can assure you that is not the case. There are millions of women, worldwide, who are all searching for answers.

I know firsthand that this search is not straightforward. Since my own personal hair loss journey began over a decade ago, I have been painstakingly researching women's hair loss, reading every bit of science I could find. I'm a former registered nurse (RN) with a burning desire to find answers and to help others. When I realised that the information available for women was sadly lacking, as was the knowledge and advice from the medical fraternity in general, I realised I had a lot of work to do.

The first time you noticed your hair loss is probably embedded in your memory, as it is for me. I remember the moment – exactly where I was and where I was sitting – when someone said that they'd noticed I was losing my hair. Until that point I had thought I was covering it with styling. But sadly, apparently not.

I recall every single moment in my early hair loss journey as if it was yesterday: the day my hair stylist pointed to a small round bald patch above my left ear that I had no idea was even there; the day on holiday in Cyprus when I pulled a fistful of hair out of my head; the gut-wrenching, sick-in-the-stomach feeling of knowing my hair was slowly but surely dwindling; and the growing worry that one day I may lose it all.

One of the hardest things about female hair loss for me initially was the lack of support available and the lack of visibility about the issue in main media, and in my everyday life from others in the same predicament. Until this happened to me, I hadn't really noticed women with hair loss. I may have seen the odd female here and there, possibly two in my whole life, but I hadn't registered it as a universal issue. And the difficulty with that is the tendency to feel very alone.

Thankfully there is now a plethora of support groups online and I'm a member of many of them. I moderate one myself. But most women who join are incredulous themselves that this is happening to them as they, like me and probably like you, had no idea that this could happen to a woman.

Unfortunately, society is quick to judge – and women tend to feel judged pretty easily. But we have to remember that we are so much more than our hair. And while we may feel that everyone is looking, they are probably not.

I imagine, like me, you took to the internet in the hunt for answers – I'm sure you can relate to endless Google searching. Unfortunately, back in 2008 when this all began for me, I found that the answers I was looking for were frustratingly lacking. Hair loss in **men** dominated the information landscape. Hair loss in **women**, although acknowledged, was sorely lacking in research and advice, and in fact, still is.

During my many hours of research, I did discover that hair loss is a rapidly rising phenomenon in women. I discovered that women all over the world were suffering from thinning hair, yet almost all of the research was on men. Even the cosmetic solutions available were almost exclusively for men.

This intrigued me: where else have we seen a cosmetic for men with no female equivalent? Surely other women felt as I did. I needed an aesthetic solution for my thinning hair so that I could feel confident while I continued to search for answers. And opening my bathroom cupboard to take out a men's hair loss product every day was not going to do it for me.

For many women, hair loss has crushed their confidence, creating social isolation and avoidance due to a deep embarrassment. As a former RN I am astutely aware of the substantial psychosocial impact of hair loss on women and the damage this can do to a woman's self-esteem. With many years in medical marketing and as an entrepreneur, and with the understanding from my own personal lived experience, I felt I needed to demystify this largely misunderstood condition and learn as much as I could about female hair loss. I had a deep desire to help women understand this condition while doing all I could to find the answers. At the same time, I needed to make an immediate cosmetic solution available **for women.**

By 2013 the findings of my independent research had become a popular women's hair loss blog.[1] I had developed a range of cosmetic products designed specifically for women to provide an instant aesthetic solution to the problem, and by 2016 I had written my first book on the topic.[2]

In the years since, I have continued my research and have learnt so much more. I have much to share with you.

If you are feeling rejected by doctors who believe there is nothing they can do, or who want to prescribe medication you are unsure about, then let me assure you, there are answers here in my book for you.

You may have bought this book to help educate yourself on the loss of your once-healthy hair. You may have lost your hair gradually or suddenly or perhaps you've never had a mane of thick, healthy hair and you're looking for ways to improve your hair health. In this book you will discover there are many factors and causes involved in poor hair health and female hair loss. I believe there is never just one cause at play; there is almost always **more than one cause operating at any one time**. I wrote this book to help you get to the bottom of the causes of your hair loss, and to guide you in creating a strategy for improving it.

As you will read at various points in this book, I have most of my hair back now – **not** due to an expensive supplement, miracle oil, spray or potion or any other product I am going to convince you to buy – so you can rest easy on that!

My hair is much thicker than it was 10 years ago due to an increased understanding of the causes of my hair loss and a consistent commitment to rectifying those.

I am going to share with you firsthand what can be done.

So let's get into it.

YOUR QUESTIONS ANSWERED

Like me you probably have many questions...

- Why me?
- What has caused this?
- Is this permanent?
- Will it get worse?
- What can I do about it?

The answers are all in this book. I have read hundreds of scientific research papers and journal articles (see Notes section at the end of the book) and fielded thousands of questions about hair loss from women of all ages and from all over the globe.

My investigations point to some new thinking around female hair loss and its causes, and I sincerely hope the topics covered here provide some clarity and relief for you in your own hair loss journey.

It is widely understood that hair loss in women is both:

- *polygenic* – meaning that it can be influenced by more than one gene, and
- *multifactorial* – meaning there are usually several factors involved in its development.

This makes the quest for solving the mystery of female hair loss very challenging, indeed! It is little wonder doctors who are not specialists in this field are unable to pinpoint the reasons women are losing hair.

Before you begin exploring the information outlined in this book, I'd like to emphasise three main ideas about female hair loss that I believe can contribute to an improved understanding of the phenomena in general:

1. There are many underlying **causes** and **triggers** for female hair loss – often many are at play at the same time.

2. An understanding of the difference between **cause** and **correlation** is necessary when exploring the complex issue of hair loss in women.

3. When describing hair loss in women, I prefer to use the term **female pattern hair loss** (FPHL) rather than female androgenic alopecia (AGA), a term I see being mistakenly used as a catch-all for female hair loss.

Allow me to explain these ideas further to prepare you for absorbing the information in this book, and offer ideas on how you can apply what you learn to your unique circumstances:

UNDERLYING CAUSES AND TRIGGERS

Here is the bottom line – the causes, triggers and treatment of female hair loss are different for every woman and based on a variety of factors. I cannot emphasise enough that one of the main challenges of managing FPHL is discovering your unique root causes and triggers. It requires patience, consistent effort and seemingly endless enquiry.

There can be multiple underlying causes that go unnoticed for many years until a final 'trigger' initiates hair loss. These triggers will only lead to an onset of hair loss in susceptible individuals, and the effect of a trigger depends on whether that individual is genetically susceptible, or experiences other underlying causes. It's complicated.

To further emphasise the complexity of this problem, let me share with you that like so many women, my own underlying causes and triggers fall broadly across a number of areas.

My initial hair loss was caused by a medication that caused a hormonal imbalance – that was my first 'trigger'. Then, over time, and compounded by early surgical menopause, I developed metabolic syndrome. I also discovered my iron was dangerously low as were a few other vitamins which are vital for healthy hair growth.

Finally, as I age, my hair follicles are miniaturising as part of a natural aging process, which will continue to thin out my hair if left unchecked.

The good news is that in the years since my original trigger, and even with subsequent bouts of hair loss caused by new triggers, I have managed to regrow my hair back each time, as well as thicken it up.

People who don't know me well, and don't know about my hair loss journey, never notice my hair loss because cosmetic camouflage (with a product I developed for just this purpose) works so well to hide it. I have also used very specific shampoos with ingredients that encourage healthy hair growth, which I needed.

In addition, it seemed with age and all the hair loss issues I've had, that new hair had stopped growing. I will share with you the ingredients in shampoos and other styling products that I used to turn that around and I'll let you know the ingredients I recommend and those to avoid.

I would like you to understand that there is not a quick fix for FPHL. If you have a bout of sudden shedding it will take time to resolve. If you have other underlying health issues contributing to your hair loss, as I have had, then you need to be consistent in your approach.

A good example of the consistency required for managing FPHL has been my daily iron and vitamin D supplementation regime. Ten years ago my levels were very low but I've now achieved levels well within the 'normal' range. This took time – it was 18 months before I could really see the benefits that supplementation had on my bloodwork and subsequently, my hair. But I was consistent and committed in my approach.

My nutritional improvement doesn't alter the fact that I also have miniaturisation due to age, but it does mean that I've minimised nutritional deficiency as a causative factor and, I believe, really slowed down the process as a result.

As you explore the ideas presented in this book and begin to make choices about which routes to take, please consider that these solutions will take time to take effect. Remember, too, that every healing strategy is just one facet of attending to the possibility of multiple causes and triggers.

CORRELATION DOES NOT IMPLY CAUSATION!

This well-known phrase refers to the inability to legitimately deduce a cause-and-effect relationship between two events or variables solely based on an association (or correlation) between them.

We can see this in action in the proliferation of social media groups focused on female hair loss, where certain factors are simply assumed to cause hair loss.

A ketogenic diet is a great example – because many women notice hair loss, possibly for the first time in their life, after a period of time on a ketogenic diet. Keto diet groups on Facebook light up the minute someone asks if any other women have noticed hair loss. But as you will read later on when I cover ketogenic diets in full, at best, that change in diet and weight loss could be a trigger. However, as not everyone on a keto diet loses their hair, it is not a simple case that keto diets cause hair loss. That's correlation not cause.

As another example, numerous studies have shown that women taking hormone replacement therapy (HRT) had a lower than average incidence of coronary heart disease (CHD), leading doctors to propose that HRT was protective against CHD. This (faulty) conclusion is often used in support of HRT to this day.

However, in some later trials it became clear that taking HRT led to a small but statistically significant increase in the risk of CHD.[3] A reanalysis of the data from the original studies showed that women undertaking HRT were more likely to be from higher socioeconomic groups with above average diet and exercise regimens and lifestyle habits. Further studies have confirmed that the benefits of a healthy diet and exercise demonstrates a significant benefit for CHD risk in healthy women initiating oestrogen therapy soon after the onset of menopause.[4] Thus, the use of HRT and the decreased incidence of coronary heart disease were *coincident effects* of a common cause.

Correlation, not causation

To illustrate the point (but in a slightly more amusing way), let's consider the strong correlation between the number of people who have died falling into a swimming pool and the number of movies that Nicholas Cage has been in, seen in the chart below.

You'll clearly see that there is a strong correlation between these two sets of data. But of course, the correlation in this case does not equal causation. We know that logically, without needing to further analyse the data. It's just logic!

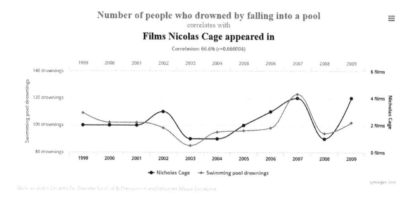

The knowledge that correlation does not imply causation is not new. However, over the past decade of thoroughly researching women's hair loss, I have noticed a very strong reliance on correlations in trying to make sense of this difficult and complex phenomenon.

Naturally, women want to know *why* they are losing their hair. We feel that if we can figure out what is causing our hair loss, we're on the way to finding a 'cure'. We want a linear path where we find, treat, reverse and fix the cause to achieve the cure. But the reality is never this clear cut.

This is also true when it comes to solutions. Switching shampoo or taking a supplement or putting oil drops on your scalp, do not stop hair falling out immediately and do not cause hair to grow miraculously in a month. Those are coincidental effects.

Male pattern balding (MPB) is much more thoroughly understood than FPHL. I believe there are two reasons for this. The majority of research into MPB has been undertaken by men, who are so visibly and obviously affected by it in very large numbers. This has resulted in a great deal of resources, time, money and effort being put into understanding the mechanisms and causes. Additionally, there appears to be a more straightforward biological pathway to the development of hair loss in men.

Put simply, it's easier to understand hair loss in men than it is in women.

By contrast, FPHL is an extremely complex issue affecting women of all ages and socioeconomic groups, all races and ethnicities (some more than others) and all levels of health, with few common links identified to date.

This is why it's so important to understand the difference between cause and correlation.

As you read this book, you'll see that there are many possible causes of female hair loss. But I believe there is never just one cause at play in any person at any one time. I believe there is an unique set of factors operating at any one time for every woman experiencing hair loss.

FEMALE PATTERN HAIR LOSS (FPHL) VS ANDROGENIC ALOPECIA

Androgenic alopecia (or *androgenetic alopecia* which is another name for the same thing) is so called because in male pattern hair loss, the cause is most often the conversion of testosterone (an androgenic hormone) to dihydrotestosterone (DHT), which is taken up by the androgen receptors in the hair follicles on the scalp. This leads to a miniaturising or 'shrinking' of the follicles until hair growth stops altogether.

However, according to a clinical review published in 2008,[5] 'most women with female pattern hair loss do not demonstrate clinical or biochemical evidence of androgen excess when tested'. That is, women's hair loss is not caused by the same pathology and hormonal factors as men's hair loss.

There are many other studies which I refer to later, which also lead me to suggest that FPHL is highly unlikely to be caused by an excess of androgens, *in the majority of cases*. While it may have been a natural conclusion to draw in the absence of any other factors or data, it would appear to be inaccurate to name the phenomenon in women 'androgenic alopecia'. Doctors and medical scientists who had no idea what was causing the problem in women simply added 'female' to the established name of the male condition. Although understandable, I do believe it has been the cause of great confusion.

It has also, unfortunately, led to the very common misdiagnosis (and, therefore, treatment) of female hair loss. It's not surprising that a large number of women report no response to anti-androgen treatments – because they're geared towards what works, hormonally, for men.

As you will see as you read on, FPHL has a long list of possible causes and triggers. Unfortunately, it is not just a simple case of too much of one particular hormone on the scalp. If only it were that simple.

TIME AND PERSEVERANCE

Due to the time involved in the hair growth cycle and the phases of 'growth, pause, shed and regrow', and the potential for a complicated mesh of various factors, it takes a long time to remedy any kind of female hair loss situation – sometimes years.

Whether it's changing shampoos and hair products, taking nutritional or herbal supplements or other strategies, a month or two is simply not long enough to deduce whether they are having a positive effect. Perseverance is key: your strategy could be working very well but it will take time to see the results. Ongoing commitment to the lifelong management of your hair loss is a part of this journey.

There is no foolproof cure for female hair loss. But there are plenty of ways to stop its progression. The younger you are and the faster you attend to your hair loss, the better your outcome will be.

One of the most common types of hair loss in women is *telogen effluvium* (TE), a fast and furious shedding of hair that is very noticeable when washing your hair due to hair building up in the drain, an abundance of hair on your brush and sometimes, hair noticeably falling out during the day. This kind of hair loss can resolve itself over time. I explain TE in full in a section devoted to it.

In my case and I believe for most other women, TE occurs due to an identifiable trigger, of which there are many. What is interesting is that the same trigger doesn't affect everyone. So there is something else going on. It's not just the trigger that is at play – there are other underlying causes as I've already mentioned.

The information in this book will help you not only to figure out your trigger but also to identify other factors that have contributed to the trigger taking effect, which will help to ensure that your hair health improves over the longer term so that future triggering events don't cause a TE response.

A QUICK NOTE ON SUPPLEMENTS

I will stress again and again throughout this book that taking a supplement of a nutrient that you are not deficient in, and therefore don't need, must never be done, especially without medical supervision. Please don't begin taking a supplement because it helped another woman without investigating your own situation with a doctor.

Many supplements can even cause or worsen hair loss when taken in high and unnecessary doses.

Although I am a former RN with many years' experience and specific knowledge gained from 13 years of researching and writing about female hair loss, as well as from thousands of comprehensive discussions with women suffering this phenomenon, I don't know your personal medical history. I don't know what medications you are taking and I don't know your specific causes or triggers. My advice should not be taken as medical advice and at no point should you ignore, or avoid, your doctor's advice in favour of mine.

However I can promise you one thing: you will discover information in this book that seems like a complete revelation, and you'll have more than one 'aha' moment! If you stick with it – learning about FPHL and building your therapeutic strategy – your hair and scalp health will thank you and you will see brighter days.

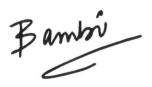

ABBREVIATIONS USED IN THIS BOOK

AE	anagen effluvium
AGA	androgenic alopecia
ANB	alternate nostril breathing
CDC	Centre for Disease Control
CHD	coronary heart disease
CTE	chronic telogen effluvium
DEA	cocamide diethanolamine
DHT	dihydrotestosterone
DMDM	DMDM hydantoin
FDA	Food and Drug Administration
FFA	frontal fibrosing alopecia
FPHL	female pattern hair loss
FUE	follicular unit extraction

FUT	follicular unit transplant
HRT	hormone replacement therapy
IBS	irritable bowel syndrome
LLLT	low-level laser therapy
MEA	cocamide monoethanolamine
MPB	male pattern balding
PCOS	polycystic ovarian syndrome
PRP	platelet-rich plasma
RN	registered nurse
SPF	sun protection factor
TE	telogen effluvium
TGA	Therapeutic Goods Administration
UV	ultraviolet

Part I

Understanding the basics

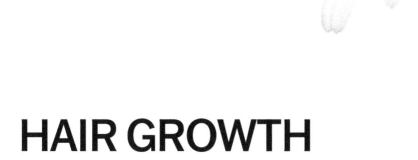

HAIR GROWTH AND HAIR LOSS

The key to understanding hair loss lies in understanding the normal hair growth cycles. Let's begin with the biological basics.

The human body grows three different types of hair:

- vellus hair
- lanugo hair
- terminal hair

Vellus hair is the fine, downy hair (aka 'peach fuzz') that covers most of our body. Although it's usually almost invisible, it may be more visible on some people than others and may increase in visibility during puberty. Its function is to help regulate our body temperature.

Lanugo hair is the fine 'fur' that covers babies in utero. Once a baby is born, lanugo hair becomes vellus hair. In some cases lanugo hair may reappear later in life. For example, individuals with anorexia nervosa, or who become drastically underweight or malnourished for other reasons, often regrow lanugo hair.

Terminal hair is the hair type we're concerned about in this book. Terminal hair is the hair on our heads, genitals, underarms and some other areas and it grows in distinct cycles. When these cycles are disrupted, affected or changed, we can experience hair loss. The function of terminal hair growth cycles in each individual can be influenced by many different variables, including genetics.

HAIR GROWTH CYCLES

Hair growth is cyclical, passing through three main phases:[6]

- anagen (the growth phase)
- catagen (the rest phase)
- telogen (the shedding phase).

Anagen phase

The anagen or 'growth' phase lasts between two and six years, depending largely on genetics. Each new hair that grows replaces a previously shed hair. This occurs approximately three months after the old hair was shed.

It is interesting to note that some ethnic groups naturally have a longer anagen phase than others. You may have seen 'miracle' hair growth products hailing from remote tribal communities where all the women and children have hair length past the waist, with gleam and shine. This is not due to the miracle product they're selling, but thanks to their genetic lottery win.

During the anagen phase, the cells in the root of each individual strand of hair quickly divide, and each hair will grow at the average rate of around one centimetre every 28 days. Interestingly, hair grows faster in summer than in winter.

Catagen phase

The catagen, or 'resting', phase lasts for several weeks after the anagen phase is complete.

During this time, the hair follicle 'shrinks', and cuts the hair off from its blood supply. The follicle then pushes the disconnected hair closer to the surface of the skin as the follicle renews itself.

Telogen phase

The telogen, or 'shedding', phase can last anywhere from one to four months.

During this phase, some hairs remain anchored to the follicle while others fall out. At any one time, around 15% of your hair is in the telogen phase – these are the hairs you lose when you brush or wash your hair. Approximately three months after a hair has been shed, the follicle will re-enter the anagen phase, recommencing the cycle.

Depending on the type of hair loss you're experiencing, the cycle is affected either temporarily or permanently. For example, in hereditary hair loss, this cycle can become a lot faster and it may take only months for a new hair to be shed. In other cases, a new hair may not replace the recently shed hair at all.

NORMAL HAIR LOSS

No-one, whether male or female, has the hair at age 50 that they had in their teens. Hair loss, thinning and gradual miniaturisation of the follicles are all a natural part of ageing. It is perfectly normal and natural to experience some thinning hair with age.

Of course, there are degrees of thinning and for women any amount of thinning can be a concern. If you are young and you have noticeable hair loss, then it may feel even more distressing. Unless we have older female relatives or friends with hair loss, most women have no idea that it's even a possibility for them. Men assume that they could, or probably will, one day lose their hair, but women do not.

While you will read in other literature that it is considered 'normal' to lose anywhere from 50 to 150 hairs a day, I question this and believe that everyone's 'normal' is different.

These days I lose much less than 50 hairs on an average day. When I wash my hair I am aware of less than 10 hairs in the shower. There may be another couple when I blow dry my hair with a round brush, but that's all.

One hundred hairs a day would be abnormal and concerning for me. You will know what is normal for you and you will be able to determine if your level of hair loss is abnormal for you.

Earlier I referred to the normal cycles of hair growth and fall. Since all hair goes through these cycles, including dormant stages followed by fall, it makes sense that some hair will be falling out every day. It's a perfectly normal process.

But, especially for women who have longer hair, a pile of hair in one 'bunch' can look like a severe and sudden loss. You may have seen images posted on Facebook or other social media, showing a pile of shed hair, shared by women who are extremely concerned about the excessive quantity. And for good reason.

Shed hair and especially if it's long, can look quite overwhelming when it's 'piled up' like this. Especially when it is an unusual amount for that woman.

Whether it's 10 hairs a day or 100, it's important to know your own baseline 'normal' for hair loss.

Seasonal hair loss

According to research from the United Kingdom,[7] many women experience seasonal hair loss. That is, there are specific times of year when more hair noticeably falls out than at other times. You may experience this yourself; I certainly do.

I was in my early 40s when I first became aware of an unusual amount of hair loss. I decided to track it in my diary as I had a suspicion that the same thing had happened before. I wondered if it was seasonal. Sure enough, the same thing happened a year later. For me it was in autumn (or . . . fall!) that I noticed significantly increased loss.

Seasonal hair loss could be a sign of things to come, as it was in my case. Or it may be quite mild and nothing to be concerned about. My suggestion is to observe and keep track when you start noticing unusual, or increased, hair loss. If you begin to notice patterns throughout the year, these ebbs and flows of hair loss may show themselves to be perfectly normal and healthy for you, or they may highlight problems.

Hair washing and brushing

It is normal and healthy for a certain amount of hair to be lost during washes, but many women find their hair loss seemingly increasing when they wash it. This can understandably lead to hair washing avoidance as a prevention strategy. Unfortunately this will invariably lead to greater frustration since not washing your hair doesn't yield the results you want.

All day, every day, there are some strands of hair that are in the fall stage that don't fall out until you brush or wash your hair. The longer you wait between washes or brushes, the more hairs there will be in the fall stage, so you will feel you have experienced a sudden loss. When in fact you haven't.

It is certainly true that over washing, washing in excessively hot water and/or using harsh chemicals on the hair can cause it to dry out and break more easily. Here is where good quality products and washing techniques really matter.

I cover this in later chapters, where I also recommend the best types of shampoo, conditioner and ingredients to help manage thinning hair.

TYPES OF HAIR LOSS

The types of hair loss covered in this book fall into two main categories:

- shedding
- gradual hair loss.

These are the main types of unexpected female hair loss that baffle women and doctors everywhere.

Shedding or hair fall (called *telogen effluvium* or TE) is very obvious for a number of reasons. You may notice hair clogging the shower drain, handfuls of hair coming out when washing, hair on the pillow in the morning or a larger than usual amount of hair coming away when brushing or running your fingers through your hair. This kind of hair loss is usually temporary.

Gradual hair loss, as the name suggests, happens over time. As each hair is shed, as part of the normal hair growth cycle, a new hair replaces it. Gradual hair loss is the process of miniaturisation of the diameter of the hair shaft. As each new hair grows to replace the previously shed hair, the new hair is narrower than the old hair.

Over time, and if not treated in any way, this will continue until eventually the miniaturised hair is so fine, it doesn't grow at all.

There is plenty written about this type of hair loss associated with the natural process of ageing.[8] But it is when this happens much earlier in a woman's life, that it is both unexpected and very worrying.

In some women this kind of thinning can initially look like hair has been lost, especially for women with very thick, coarse hair. In fact, the hair is still there and the follicle is still sending up a new hair, but the follicle is in the process of miniaturisation. Many women who have naturally thick hair strands may first notice that they can see their scalp through their hair. This is because there appears to be a greater distance between each, now finer, hair, which is especially evident in women with dark hair.

There are many different ways in which this kind of hair loss can present.

When miniaturisation and progressive hair loss occurs as part of the aging process, it is the cells that feed the hair follicle which deteriorate.

This kind of hair loss can also happen at a much earlier age. In fact, it can be happening without a woman having any idea that the process is taking place.

As described later in this book, there are many causes of a deterioration in hair diameter and quantity, and/or a disruption to the growth cycles: from nutritional deficiencies to medications (some of which can cause hair loss and can even contribute to nutritional deficiencies), to hormonal changes, to metabolic disorders and genetic factors. The mechanisms behind this broad range of causes are part of the reason that figuring out how to resolve female hair loss is so difficult.

One sign of miniaturisation is a change in the quality of the hair itself.

As the diameter of the hair follicle miniaturises, the hair shaft becomes finer, and is often curlier and frizzier. Many women gradually come to the realisation that humidity now has a negative effect on their hair, where it once did not, as it becomes an unsightly mass of frizz. These changes in hair texture can be the first sign of gradual miniaturisation.

Of course, these changes can occur in any order. You may have had a bout of shedding, followed by regrowth, followed by something else that triggers another bout of shedding.

Then over time you realise that your hair texture and volume has changed.

This could mean that each time your hair grew back, the diameter was slightly smaller – a situation where miniaturisation coincides with shedding. So, both types of hair loss could be happening at the same time.

How do we begin to figure out what is going on in our body and not just *what* but of course, as every woman wants to know, *why*. I believe that there is always an underlying cause or causes and a trigger.

Some underlying causes may be gradually working away at the miniaturisation process, while others may not be having any effect. Some underlying causes may never result in hair loss, yet others may. It all depends on a combination of factors and whether or not there is a trigger.

While genetics do play a role in hair loss in women, it isn't clear exactly how. There is one theory that the genetic potential may remain a dormant weakness that never eventuates. But that if triggered, it may.

We can't simply assume that what was a trigger in one person will be a trigger for another. We can't assume that an underlying cause in someone else will be the same for us. And we can't assume that because a female in your genetic line has hair loss that you will – nor if no-one does, that you won't.

This really is a difficult subject to navigate.

The further you read, the more I hope to help you figure out and get clear on your underlying causes and potential triggers.

Alopecia

Alopecia is the medical term for hair loss. No matter what type of hair loss you have, or its cause, you technically have alopecia.

The term comes from a Greek word meaning 'fox', a creature that sheds its hair all year round.

If you hear this word as part of a medical diagnosis, there's no cause for panic – it does not necessarily mean that you will become completely bald. There are a few different forms of alopecia and their clinical features vary depending on the type of hair loss and the cause.

Alopecia areata

Alopecia areata is an autoimmune disease which can present in many forms:

- patchy hair loss all over the scalp (*alopecia areata*)
- complete baldness of the scalp (*alopecia totalis*)
- baldness in one area of the scalp (*alopecia areata monolocularis*)
- hair loss in multiple areas (*alopecia areata multilocularis*)
- total hair loss: head, face, body, pubic hair etc. (*alopecia universalis*).

Areas of hair loss in people with alopecia areata are usually well defined, rounded patches. Like most autoimmune diseases, the condition occurs due to the body's inability to differentiate between its own cells and foreign cells. This leads to the body attacking its own cells, in this case, the anagen hair follicles. Alopecia areata is quite rare (affecting 0.1–0.2% of people) so it's unlikely to be the reason for your hair loss. However, you are more likely to have alopecia areata if you have a family history of it, or have other autoimmune diseases.

Thoroughly examine the patterns of your hair loss and if you notice your hair loss is occurring in well-defined, circular patches, you **may** have alopecia areata. Visit your doctor for a professional opinion who may refer you to a specialist.

If it is determined that alopecia areata is the reason for your hair loss, don't fret. Often the condition will fix itself within a few months to a year. There are also medications (most commonly corticosteroids) that you can take to speed up the return of your hair. You may get flare-ups from time to time, especially during periods of stress, so it's important to understand your own causes and manage your triggers as best as you can.

I can speak from personal experience here, as I experienced alopecia areata some years before my first telogen effluvium (TE). One day my hairdresser pointed out that there was a complete bald patch on the side of my head above my left ear. I didn't fret about it as it was hidden from view and, to be honest, I completely forgot about it. It resolved itself within a few months.

However, this did herald a future of battling hair loss for me.

Female pattern hair loss (FPHL)

Female hair loss can be patchy, patterned or diffuse:

- Patchy is generally seen in well-defined patches just as it sounds.
- Patterned tends to occur in a set pattern usually beginning with a widening part.
- Diffuse refers to a more generalised hair loss dispersed or spread out all over the scalp.

Female hair loss is often referred to as *androgenic alopecia (AGA)*. However, scientists are increasingly questioning the use of the term 'androgenic' when describing female hair loss[9].

The use of the term 'androgenic' in the name refers to the aetiology or the pathological process from which the outcome stems.

Male hair loss has been known since antiquity. In 400 BCE Hippocrates observed that eunuchs did not develop baldness. In 1942, James B Hamilton noted (through extensive studies on male pattern baldness and observing the lack of hair loss in eunuchs) that the male androgen hormones, including testosterone, were involved.[10]

Androgenic alopecia therefore became the most widely used term to describe male pattern baldness. Once doctors started seeing hair loss in women, and with no clue as to why it was happening, it appears that both doctors and scientists alike assumed the aetiology was the same. Hence, they adopted the term '*female* androgenic alopecia' to describe female hair loss.

Androgenic alopecia begins with testosterone at the hair follicle. Testosterone, circulating in the blood stream, is taken up in the follicle and converted to dihydrotestosterone (DHT) by an enzyme called 5a-reductase. The more 5areductase someone has, the more DHT will be created in that conversion process. And it is DHT which acts on the follicle to cause it to deteriorate, thin out and eventually not grow.

While women also have these hormones and enzymes in their bodies, the amount of it and its actions on the scalp and the hair follicles do not appear to be the same.

According to a review published in 2015, 'while the follicular changes that lead to alopecia are similar between men and women, clinical presentation and response to antiandrogen therapy are different'.[11] In other words, women don't tend to respond to the androgenic hormonal treatments given to men.

An earlier article, published in 1999, discussed the case of a young woman with what appeared to be the clinical presentation of female androgenic alopecia but with an absence of circulating androgens, indicating that her pattern hair loss was not androgen dependent.[12]

Given the young age of some of the women with female pattern hair loss, it does appear that it would be both incorrect and unhelpful to simply describe all pattern female hair loss as 'androgenic'. And in my view, without this distinction, research will not adequately advance, and women will continue to be treated with the same medications that work for men.

For this reason, female pattern hair loss (FPHL) is the term I use to describe female hair loss and the term I use throughout this book.

FPHL is usually characterised by non-scarring (which means that the hair follicle has remained intact), diffuse hair loss or alopecia. 'Diffuse' refers to the pattern of hair loss, being spread out, in contrast to alopecia areata mentioned previously where the hair loss occurs in one patch. FPHL usually occurs in the front, the top of the head and through to the crown. It can occur in just one of these areas or all of them. It is often characterised by a widening of the hair part.

As previously mentioned, your hair loss will most likely fall into one of two categories. FPHL is one which will affect more than 50% of women at some stage in their lives.

Telogen effluvium

As with FPHL, *telogen effluvium* (TE) is very common and presents when your body has undergone a period of stress. This could include emotional stress, like a divorce, a major car accident or losing your job; or it could be symptomatic of physical stress like major surgery, dramatic weight loss or a severe illness. Hair growth is not a high priority for our body, so when we encounter stressful experiences our body will become strategic about managing its resources. It will cease to consider growing hair as a necessity.

You may be thinking 'This isn't me, life's good at the moment'; however, to fully understand the life and health of our hair, we need to bear in mind the nature of the hair growth cycle. It is usually around three months **after** the stress occurred, which is when your hair growth cycle was interrupted, that you notice the hair fall. The good news is, if stress-related telogen effluvium is your problem, your body should regain its equilibrium on its own and resume healthy regrowth of your hair. Later in this book I discuss the effects of stress in more detail as well as provide information about how you can better care and nourish your hair back to good health by improving and managing, not just your hair health, but also your stress levels. Recovery from a bout of TE can take a long time. I have had several bouts of TE over the years and on each occasion the recovery and regrowth has followed in different ways and for differing lengths of time.

Working on your general hair health with all the advice I offer here is a great way to ensure that your recovery from any future TE is faster and more complete. Better underlying health and optimal hair health can even help in preventing a future bout of TE. Remember, a trigger may or may not cause TE, depending on the presence of, or the lack of, underlying causes.

I have improved my hair health immeasurably and haven't had a bout of TE in nearly 5 years. I have been ill and I have had some very stressful times, but nothing has triggered TE for me, even though it was a previous tendency.

Chronic telogen effluvium

Telogen effluvium usually resolves within three to six months. When the hair loss continues beyond 6 months, it is referred to as chronic telogen effluvium (CTE).

Chronic telogen effluvium typically affects women between 30 and 50 who have a very full, thick head of hair.[13] There is often a history of having been able to grow hair very long which would indicate a long anagen phase.

CTE could indicate that the underlying causes that were present at the beginning of the TE have not been rectified. These will be covered in full later, but can be due to a medication, an iron deficiency, malabsorption, poor diet or thyroid disease and a range of other possible causes including stress. This is why I will aways advocate that women need to identify their underlying causes and work on rectifying them.

Although the prognosis is not certain, and the hair shedding follows a fluctuating course, CTE does usually resolve spontaneously, although could take as long as three to four years.[14] And women do not go bald despite having the condition.

Frontal fibrosing alopecia

Frontal fibrosing alopecia (FFA) is thought to be a form of *lichen planopilaris* and is quite rare. It is a type of hair loss that occurs around the hair line, most notably at the front, but can occur all the way around the hair line. It can also occur in the eyebrows and eyelashes, the beard in men and other parts of the body. It is a slow and progressive type of hair loss and as it occurs the follicles are no longer visible. It is known as a 'scarring' type of hair loss.

There is likely a genetic factor involved, but there can also be hormonal, autoimmune, inflammatory and environmental elements involved.

FFA tends to occur in post-menopausal women, which would point to a largely hormonal aetiology. However, there is usually more than one factor involved.

Women of African descent have a slightly different presentation to Caucasian women. Firstly, it tends to happen to them at a younger age and secondly, it is often overlooked due to the prevalence of *traction alopecia*. Traction alopecia occurs when the hair is constantly pulled back so tightly that the hair at the front is put under constant strain and the follicles eventually stop producing hair.

SCALP DISCOMFORT

If you're losing more hair than usual and it's accompanied by a sore or itchy scalp, then you should seek medical advice as you may have a scalp condition that is causing your hair to fall.

The good news is that when scalp issues are resolved, hair loss usually reverses and normal growth is re-established.

You may suspect scalp problems if you experience sensations that feel like your hair has been up in a tight ponytail for too long: each hair hurts as you move it. This seems to be a common complaint among women with scalp issues and I experience it myself from time to time.

It could be a sign of inflammation, which can also be associated with hair loss, but it could also be nothing to worry about. There are plenty of topical treatments available if it is a scalp issue, from creams to medicated shampoos.

Also, use the best low-chemical shampoos you can find and be as kind to your hair and scalp as possible.

Hair loss accompanied by other symptoms

If you notice an increase in your hair loss accompanied by feeling unwell, or simply not like your usual self, there could be other medical issues worth investigating with your doctor. Some vitamin and mineral deficiencies can cause hair loss while also causing fatigue and lethargy, and you may find that correcting them may help your hair regain strength while making you feel a whole lot better. As I'll keep repeating, it's important to establish a deficiency before taking supplements.

Hair loss can also be a symptom of other illnesses, like auto-immune diseases and thyroid disorders, so the sooner you seek medical advice the sooner you can address any health issues you may have.

Part II

Female pattern hair loss

CAUSES AND TRIGGERS

I have been researching FPHL and talking to thousands of women with hair loss for over 10 years now, and one thing has become abundantly clear . . .

Doctors struggle the world over to provide answers for women with hair loss.

This is explained by what you now know: that female hair loss is triggered by a unique set of factors and circumstances, which can be different for each woman. Further, that there are usually many causes, triggers and factors involved. No wonder doctors have little clue where to begin.

FPHL, the type of female hair loss we are talking about in this book, generally results from the combination of an underlying cause, or causes, and a trigger.

Underlying causes tend to be systemic and/or metabolic and have been occurring over a long period of time. These include factors like lowering oestrogen, low iron, poor nutrition, obesity, hypothyroidism or digestive issues.

Triggers, on the other hand, are 'events', or changes in biological circumstances, which might include factors like stress, surgery, accidents, new medications or acute illnesses or infections.

According to a recent review published in the International Journal of Women's Dermatology, hair loss in women is *polygenic* (can be influenced by more than one gene) and *multifactorial* (dependent on a number of factors) with the additional influence of environmental factors.[15]

This explains the broad range of causes for hair loss, from the obvious such as damage with peroxides and other chemicals, to 'hidden' causes, like systemic inflammation and stress. There are literally dozens of possible combinations of causes: multiply one genetic factor with a few dozen biological and environmental causes, add another genetic factor with a bunch of other elements in turn, and there is no simple answer as to why your hair is unexpectedly falling out.

As you come to understand FPHL, start to consider your own possible underlying causes, or contributing factors. Then try to identify a potential trigger. Remember there can be more than one underlying cause, as there could be more than one trigger.

You may be one of those women who has joined a social media group, hoping to find your answers with the help of other women. Please try to remember, as you engage with these online platforms and support groups, that what may be causing the problem for one woman will be different for another. This journey is about you and your individual, physiological health and lifestyle. The information I have compiled here is designed to empower you to make informed and wise choices.

And a word of warning . . . I've seen women 'prescribing' over-the-counter medications and supplements to one another online. As a health professional, it is horrifying to see women telling others to supplement or medicate with no qualification or knowledge of another's medical history.

WHEN CAUSES COMBINE

It's important to understand that it's becoming more and more evident, through research on female hair loss, that causes are rarely ever working alone. More often than not, they're working in combination.

For example, menopause is considered a common cause of hair loss for women. Indeed, it would appear to be the case from anecdotal evidence and it's something many women clearly notice.

Similarly, ketogenic diets are also commonly associated with hair loss in women. It may seem that there is a clear connection between hair loss and a keto diet for women in midlife and beyond, but it may not be quite so simple.

We need to consider the possible *conflation* of these two factors: many women in menopause adopt 'crash' diets to eliminate their menopause weight gain, and ketogenic diets are more popular than ever. Not all women lose their hair as they go through menopause, and not all women on ketogenic diets lose their hair. But *many* women report hair loss when both factors are simultaneously at play.

We know that female hair loss is multifactorial, which means there are many factors that contribute to female hair loss, so we need to keep this in mind as we aim to get to the causes of our own.

We'll look at both menopause and ketogenic diets as potential contributing factors to FPHL a little later on.

One thing we can all agree on is that doctors struggle the world over to find answers and solutions for women with hair loss. This has largely to do with each woman having a unique set of factors that have contributed to her condition. There are no 'rules' for women's hair loss.

GENETICS

Naturally our genetics play a pivotal role in our individual biological make-up.

It's a common belief that we inherit hair loss from our mother's side: the maternal line. This is largely because the gene that is responsible for baldness in men is on the X chromosome, and a male's X chromosome comes from his mother. But, in fact, hair loss can be inherited from either parent or genetic line.

This means that your mother may have hair loss and you do not, or your mother may have a mane of healthy hair while you suffer thinning and shedding. The same is true relating to your father – the paternal line. Both parent's genes have played a part in your development and tendencies. As such, your hair type and tendency to thin (or not) could come from either parent – or from both. This said, there is some evidence that for men whose father and/or grandfather and/or other close male relative is bald, there is a higher tendency for balding to affect them.[16]

There would appear to be multiple genes associated with hair loss in women. But since there are multiple underlying causes and triggers associated with female hair loss, it has been thus far impossible to pinpoint exactly which genes, and from which line, are in play.[17]

In all my research, I'm yet to find any evidence that points specifically to one or other parent, or their 'line', as the culprit for causing hair loss.

Anecdotally, I see many women with hair loss who are the only female in the family with this problem. Equally, we see many women whose female relatives are also losing hair and there seems to be a strong 'inheritance' factor.

The genetics of hair loss are complex and, I have found, quite pointless to spend too much energy on. Best to put your energy into other more productive endeavours.

STRESS

There are two types of stress that can contribute to the development of FPHL:

- **Acute stress** – the stress caused by sudden, shocking, difficult things that happen, from sudden illness to the death of a loved one.
- **Cellular stress** – a long-term degenerative process that affects many cells in the body including the cells of the hair follicle.

Many women take on too much. Full time work often in very high stress professions, plus everything else expected of women from child-bearing, to child-raising, to extended family responsibilities perhaps with ageing parents, combined with home and other pressing life issues and even for some women, adding study to their list of obligations. Combine these factors with the popularity of the contraceptive pill and its resulting hormonal effects, excessive demands on our time and, for many, a tendency to rely on a poor quality, fast-food diet, it is little wonder you find women of all ages, with all kinds of new ailments as manifestations of stress: chronic weight gain, heart disease and, of course, hair loss.

Stress appears to cause hair loss in a variety of ways. Perhaps the most significant and a common underlying cause, is inflammation, caused by the sustained increase in the body's cortisol levels – our primary stress adaption hormone.

Long-term raised cortisol levels can lead to chronic inflammation and immune system suppression, which can lead to disease, like cancer and autoimmune diseases. In addition, this 'cortisol effect', compounded by lifestyle, poor diet and stress, leads to chronic systemic inflammation.

This is a vicious cycle: stress > raised cortisol > inflammation > female hair loss > stress.

Other factors may also be at play, such as type 2 diabetes, overweight and obesity, emotional and/or physical stress, and cellular stress that affects the mitochondria (or energy station) of the hair cell.

Stress is a major factor in our modern lives, and cortisol is the hormone we release to combat it[18]. High circulating cortisol itself, without inflammation, is a known factor in hair loss and it can be measured by scalp-hair analysis. Increased levels of cortisol have been found in the scalp hair of people with hair loss, especially if they are also obese (which is considered a form of physical stress).

OXIDATIVE STRESS AND INFLAMMATION

I have a particular interest in researching hair loss at the cellular level. There is a connection between the body's response to stress and the presence of inflammation. Further, there is a connection between inflammation and poor cellular health. Poor cellular health at the follicle level leads to poor hair health.

Oxidative stress is an imbalance between the free radicals that are present in every cell and the antioxidants that are needed to neutralise those free radicals. Too many free radicals lead to oxidative or cellular stress. The relationship between oxidative stress and inflammation has been widely studied and reported.[19]

Inflammation is a complex topic as it causes many biological responses that are not necessary to understand for our purposes. What's important is understanding the association of inflammation with many diseases including viral infections, autoimmune conditions, chronic comorbid diseases and obesity. It is also associated with consumption of alcohol, smoking and a high sugar/high calorie diet.

You may have read that antioxidants work to reverse oxidative stress. But there is much debate on that topic.[20] There is a paradox at play here which suggests that the use of antioxidants prevents the body's own mechanism from neutralising free radicals – less than ideal.

The ideal approach is to work on your overall health by giving your body what it needs and removing what it doesn't. Exposure to toxic chemicals, smoking, excessive alcohol consumption, and a poor diet are factors that contribute to inflammation – which is a key contributing factor to poor cell health. Poor cell health affects the mitochondria, or energy generator, of every cell in the body, including hair follicles.

These are all things you can work on to improve by ensuring you are getting enough natural antioxidants in your diet. Fruit and vegetables play a huge role in a healthy diet as we all know, and for good reason: they're antioxidant rich.

Here is a list of foods which you should focus on consuming if you are working on reducing your oxidative stress and inflammation:

- fish and nuts
- berries
- cherries
- citrus fruit
- dark leafy vegetables
- broccoli
- carrots

- tomatoes
- olives
- garlic
- onion

You should also look to add these to your diet if you can:

- turmeric
- cinnamon
- green tea

Other advice includes exercise, avoiding harsh chemicals as much as possible (especially in and around your hair), wearing sunscreen and, of course, if your diet is rich with all of the above you won't need to consume fast food, which is best avoided if you can.

MENOPAUSE

While women are in their childbearing years, the body has a naturally protective level of oestrogen. Oestrogen is important for women for all sorts of health metrics: brain function, memory, bone density, skin suppleness, cardiovascular health and yes, hair health and quality.

From about the age of 40, oestrogen levels begin to drop and, among other things, the density of our hair begins to decline.

One of the reasons menopause is commonly linked with female hair loss is due to the associated drop in oestrogen, as with post-pregnancy, when hair loss can also occur due to a drop in oestrogen. These hormonal shifts change the density of hair as well as the health of the follicles.[21]

However, unlike postpartum hair loss, postmenopausal hair is unlikely to return to its former glory. There are many reasons why a woman on the peri-to-post menopause spectrum may be suffering hair loss.

Some women are particularly susceptible to the lowering levels of oestrogen. Some women will have lost a lot of hair following pregnancy, while others lost none. Many women find a loss of hair density following a change in their contraceptive pill regimen.

If you are someone whose hair is sensitive to oestrogen levels when you are under 40, then you may be someone who finds hair loss is triggered easily postpartum or during perimenopause and beyond.

There are other factors that may contribute to hair loss after the age of 50.

Nutritional depletion is a major problem that often comes about through a woman making many and varied efforts to address the weight gain that can take hold during menopause. This can lead to undereating, following a diet that lacks nutritional value and, sometimes, severely disordered eating. A depleted nutritional state can result in hair loss, which is strongly associated with deficiencies in iron, vitamin D and other critical vitamins and minerals.

Other possible underlying causes around the menopausal phase can include irritable bowel syndrome (IBS), low thyroid hormones, and the side effects of medications.

Some women may be in menopause, or taking medications that are known to cause or trigger hair loss, but not experience any form of hair loss, especially if they are otherwise healthy. However, if a woman has systemic inflammation then the medication or hormonal phase may trigger hair loss. This is why, when women ask online groups and forums if others have found hair loss caused by a certain medication or trigger, there will always be a number of women who have also taken that medication successfully for many years, without a hair-loss side effect.

This is a very important distinction and one I'd like you to always keep in mind. *Remember correlation does not necessarily equal causation.* One woman's cause or trigger is not necessarily another's.

If you are well past menopause and your hair is barely growing (a natural by-product of age) then fear not. Later in this book, I provide many ways to improve the healthy growth of your hair regardless of your age. I've personally tried them all too and, as I've already mentioned, these days I have much more hair than at any time in the past 10 or so years.

INSULIN RESISTANCE

Being overweight at any age is influenced by the hormone, insulin. Usually, the issue is that the body is not able to utilise the insulin it is releasing, which causes *insulin resistance*. According to Dr Jason Fung, who co-founded the Intensive Dietary Management program, it is insulin – not calories in vs calories out – that causes weight gain. This is a huge topic and one that could fill a book. In fact, the book I most highly recommend on insulin and obesity is *The Obesity Code* by Dr Jason Fung. It is extremely eye opening.[22]

Insulin resistance is also known as metabolic syndrome, pre-diabetes and syndrome x. These names are interchangeable, so if you have been diagnosed with any of these and also have hair loss, then know there is a link.

OBESITY

Obesity is commonly associated with hair loss in women, but it's important to know that it doesn't specifically *cause* FPHL.

Rather, overweight women tend to present with high insulin, insulin resistance, systemic inflammation and/or high cortisol levels, and it is these factors that can, but don't always, influence hair loss.

This is why we may see two women going through menopause, not eating a healthy diet, who are low in iron and other nutrients, compounded by IBS, Hashimoto's Disease or another autoimmune condition, and one woman struggles with hair loss and the other has no evidence of it whatsoever.

We are all individual and not everyone's body responds to the same stimuli or influences in the same manner. A woman who is only a little overweight may have chronically low iron, whereas another woman who is morbidly obese may have loads of iron, but be chronically low in vitamin D.

Surprisingly, a woman who is malnourished can be either very thin or very overweight. Malnourishment can be caused by a poor diet but it can also be the result of malabsorption, an underlying cause of hair loss due to the lack of nutrients being absorbed.

Many of these issues can be easily diagnosed and rectified, so consulting your doctor is always a good place to start when you are trying to identify your underlying causes.

SUDDEN SHOCK

Sudden shocks, whether emotional or physical, are known to trigger hair loss. They can include the death of a loved one, a severe illness (like COVID-19), an international relocation, drastic weight loss, a change in medication, major surgery and any number of life circumstances that involve sudden and overwhelming change.

What causes the body to suddenly shed 10, 20 or 100 times more hair in response to shocks like these?

Remember the hair growth cycle? The first part is the anagen (growth) phase, which can go on for many years. Genetics and some heredity factors will determine how long your hair will grow for. Once the growing stage is over, hair enters into the second, catagen (resting) phase. This is where the hair follicle stops growing and prepares to fall out in the telogen (shedding) phase. Once shed, a new hair grows in its place some months later and the cycle begins again.

A healthy body manages the hair growth cycle, and a multitude of other bodily functions, seamlessly through every minute of the day and night. But when the body is sent into a state of sudden or prolonged shock, the mechanisms that contribute to a healthy hair growth cycle tend to receive the signal to stop the growth phase and rest. This allows the rest of the body to survive the shock by freeing up energy and resources. The body can concentrate on cell regeneration in critical areas – such as the brain, heart and lungs – by diverting energy and resources away from hair growth.

Then, the large proportion of the hairs in the growth cycle that were moved into the resting phase will fall out around three months later. This is called telogen effluvium (TE) or diffuse shedding as we explored earlier.

Hair loss doesn't happen to everyone who has surgery, loses a loved one or experiences another form of shock. Why to some and not others? The answer is in the presence of one or more underlying causes or chronic health factors.

Underlying causes are many, varied and often multiple. I've mentioned, for example, the insulin resistance often present in obese women, which can be associated with elevated cortisol and systemic inflammation. If we add in low iron, zinc or a lack of other vitamins resulting from poor dietary choices or poor absorption, we see a cocktail of causation.

That's why female hair loss can be such a mystery.

PREGNANCY

The hormonal changes in pregnancy are completely normal and required in the course of growing a human being. One of the most profound changes is the increase in oestrogen levels that is sustained throughout pregnancy. One of the side effects of the increase is a cessation or a slowing down of the hair growth/loss cycle. Many pregnant women comment on their luscious, thick hair when pregnant, only to find following birth, when the oestrogen levels drop back to normal levels, that the hair moves into the shedding phase and falls out. This is a very common process and no need for concern.

However, in some women, especially those with naturally fine or thin hair, or for someone who has had a previous bout of TE, this post-pregnancy hair loss can be quite distressing. When a woman worries consistently about the negative impact of sudden and unexpected hair loss, hair loss can increase.

This cycle of stress confirms that worry about hair loss can contribute to further hair loss[23].

Worrying about hair loss while nurturing a totally dependent infant, being sleep deprived and potentially skipping proper meals makes a woman's body vulnerable to further hair loss and thinning. It is a vicious cycle.

The good news is that most women find that their hair growth returns to normal after the postpartum phase, although this can take up to a year. Some women find that they go through this experience with all of their pregnancies, while others can be on their third or fourth pregnancy before experiencing it for the first time.

Unfortunately for others, the stress–hair loss cycle that can be triggered following pregnancy initiates a lifelong battle, setting off contributing factors that have been dormant but are revealed through pregnancy.

CONTRACEPTIVE PILL

Many women report hair loss after coming off, or changing, their contraceptive pill. The pill contains oestrogen which protects the hair, so coming off it will decrease the amount of oestrogen in the body. Some women are particularly sensitive to this oestrogen effect and may notice a hair shed when they cease taking it.

It's interesting to note that women up to the age of around 40 have the highest oestrogen levels they will ever have in their life and it is at this time that their hair will be the best it will ever be. At around 40, at the beginning of peri-menopause and beyond, oestrogen levels start to fall and hair growth will begin to decline.

For a woman whose hair was particularly sensitive to coming off oestrogen after ceasing the pill at some time in her life, this decline in oestrogen with increasing age is also likely to result in hair loss. Ageing hair loss presents as a gradual miniaturisation and is progressive.

POLYCYSTIC OVARIAN SYNDROME (PCOS)

Polycystic ovarian syndrome (PCOS) is a common underlying cause of hair loss in women that is not always otherwise evident or symptomatic. PCOS hair loss is caused by an excess of androgens – the same thing that causes men to lose their hair. Testosterone is broken down to dihydrotestosterone (DHT) which binds to a receptor in the hair follicle and gradually kills it off.

Spironolactone is a medication that is often prescribed for PCOS hair loss as it is a 'DHT blocker' and so it can prevent the hair follicle from being susceptible to DHT.

Women with PCOS are often also found to have an under-active thyroid (hypothyroidism) which is another cause of increased androgens. These are both known to cause hair loss in women.

In addition, many women with PCOS also have insulin resistance (a precursor to type 2 diabetes). Insulin resistance is one of the underlying causes identified as having the potential to cause female hair loss on its own, without the added complication of PCOS.

There are some natural ways to treat PCOS, for example with a non-inflammatory diet, reduced stress and improved gut health. Completely removing all forms of sugar from the diet is also important, especially for insulin resistance.

If you have any or all of these underlying causes they will need to be rectified before you will see any improvement in hair health. And making these diet and lifestyle changes will help hair loss whether caused by PCOS or not.

In the treatments section of this book you will see that improving general health has a huge effect on hair loss for a variety of reasons.

EXTREME WEIGHT CHANGES

Restrictive diets of all types can result in inadequate intake of various essential nutrients which, in turn, can cause hair loss.

Rapid weight loss can also cause stress and a certain level of shock to the body, which can trigger hair loss also.

Steer clear of fad diets unless you want to lose more than just weight. If weight loss is your goal, then a slow and steady loss of 500g (approximately one pound) per week is considered medically safe and unlikely to trigger hair loss.

Similarly, gaining a significant amount of weight in a short period is a significant biological stressor, and may cause hair to thin. If you need to gain weight, slow and steady is the key.

MEDICATION

Being prescribed a medication often indicates that a person is unwell, and the condition, or the stress on the body of the illness, may be causing hair loss.

But in some cases it could be the medication itself that's causing hair loss.

There are many medications that are known to cause hair loss as a side effect. These include prescriptions for blood pressure management, acne, arthritis, gout, arrhythmias and psoriasis. Further, some antifungal, anticonvulsive, antacids and steroid medications can cause hair loss too.

Check with your doctor or specialist and carefully read the package labels and inserts of your prescribed medications to determine whether their use has been associated with hair loss as a side effect.

It is also important not to overlook those medications you have been taking long term, like hormone replacement therapy (HRT) or contraceptives. Has the dosage of your medication changed? Have you recently stopped taking a medication? All of these factors can cause biological changes that can contribute to hair loss.

ILLNESS AND COVID-19

There is growing evidence that infection with COVID-19 can trigger hair loss (TE) in some women. According to an article in *The Lancet* some 10.4% of patients with confirmed COVID-19 suffered hair loss along with a variety of other long-term side effects.[24]

Acute TE has been associated with many viral infections including dengue fever, influenza, HIV, typhoid fever, scarlet fever, pneumonia, tuberculosis, pertussis and malaria. [25]

As we have seen, the hair growth cycle is viewed by the body as largely non-essential, so during illness it can be one of the first processes the body stops assigning resources to, which can result in hair loss. In fact, hair loss is a common symptom of many illnesses, especially those with autoimmune involvement.

It may surprise you to learn that even acute illnesses or infections, like gastroenteritis, can put enough stress on the body to initiate hair loss. This type of hair loss will usually amend itself without intervention as the illness resolves.

Loss of taste and smell is recognised as one of the first likely symptoms of the Delta variant of COVID-19, and some of the final symptoms to resolve, sometimes only many months after recovery. These are not the only long-lasting impacts of COVID-19. We are beginning to understand more of the long-term effects of this virus on patients who have recovered as time unfolds.

A recent study published in *The Lancet* investigated the longer-term medical impacts of COVID-19 in patients 6 months after they had contracted the disease.[26] The study showed that 81% of patients were still suffering some symptoms as a result of contracting the virus: what we now know as 'long COVID'.

Fatigue and smell loss or distortion, alongside heart palpitations and difficulty sleeping, were all prevalent in the study participants. Interestingly, the second highest reported long-COVID symptom was hair loss. In fact, the study found that one in four COVID-19 patients report hair loss months after contracting the virus, with women statistically more likely to experience this symptom.

How could this be explained?

Doctors have suggested that the hair loss experienced and reported by COVID-19 patients is not caused by the virus 'attacking' the hair follicles. Rather, it is likely a reaction caused by the physical and emotional stress brought on by the disease.

Well-known personalities have even taken to social media to show their own experience with hair loss following recovery from COVID-19. One celebrity documented large clumps of hair coming out of her hair as she brushed.

There's no doubt that contracting COVID-19 and many other viruses can cause stress on the body. But it's important to factor in many of the other aspects of living through a pandemic. We have all been living through some extremely tough times. Disruption, stress and anxiety have been a universal experience.

If COVID-19 was a hair loss trigger for you, instead of obsessing over your hair line and constantly checking to see if there's any new growth, as hard as it seems to achieve, please do try to relax about it. Remember that the stress of hair loss contributes to more hair loss. One way to reduce the stress on your self-esteem is to use a cosmetic product like Boost N Blend, a product designed for women to conceal thinning areas. These cotton fibres are a cosmetic solution and can be easily applied every day to boost confidence, while working on the underlying cause for hair loss or waiting for the post-viral symptom to resolve. The tiny fibres in these products cling to the hair shaft, making them appear thicker and fuller. This way no-one has to know that your hair changed at all during COVID-19.

And finally, rest assured, post COVID-19 hair loss does resolve in the majority of cases. Especially with no other under-lying causes in play.

In a later section of this book I review shampoos and styling products, including the ingredients to avoid and which ones to use to improve your hair health and give it the best chance of recovery.

KETOGENIC DIETS

There are lots of reasons women decide to go on a ketogenic diet, and they are especially popular among menopausal women. This is, I believe, because they are promoted to menopausal women who are frustrated with the inability to lose weight due to age and, likely, high insulin. 'Keto' diets are known to have many additional benefits, like lowering inflammation, slowing the ageing process and treating chronic illnesses.

But ketosis, the metabolic state achieved by eating a very high fat and low carbohydrate diet, when combined with a lack of sufficient protein, can act as a trigger for hair loss in susceptible individuals.

The truth is that any restrictive diet can lead to a lack of the vitamins and minerals required for healthy hair growth. Keto hair loss usually occurs due to the unhappy and untimely coinciding of underlying contributing factors, such as insulin resistance or menopause, in combination with the effects of the diet, which we can consider a trigger. The keto diet alone is not likely to cause hair loss in an otherwise healthy individual without any underlying causative factors.

Remember correlation, not causation.

COPING WITH HAIR LOSS

As you continue to learn about the causes of hair loss, keep a look out for your own possible underlying causes, which will most likely be your own unique combination of contributing factors. Then, try to identify your potential triggers. Remember there can be more than one underlying cause as there could be more than one trigger.

You hear of women who take iron supplements and their hair grows back. Then you hear of a woman who changed her shampoo and her hair grew back. But there are equally as many, if not more, women for whom those steps achieved no improvements.

Don't be disheartened. We are working through all the possible underlying causes, and you are learning how to pinpoint them and also how to identify many of the common triggers. Later I will discuss general hair health. You can then combine all the knowledge from these areas, decide what applies to you, and work towards enjoying more abundant and healthier hair for the long term.

Bear in mind that stopping the 'dreaded shed', reversing hair loss and signalling the body to grow more hair, takes time. Due to the long hair growth cycle, it is not an overnight process. But it is most definitely possible. When I originally lost my hair, it took 18 months before I saw the fruits of my labour. I persevered every day, and for many years it has been a continued priority for me. Caring for my hair health is now a ritual of self-care and a wise investment in my wellbeing.

This book is all about understanding female hair loss. Once you understand why this is happening to you and you have identified your why, you can begin the work on healing and turning your hair growth back on.

There is a lot that you can do to increase your confidence while you navigate this terrain. For a widening part, visible scalp or a balding crown, cotton hair fibres are your friend (see page 174).

Wigs and toppers (page 143) are readily available online and in stores, for managing more advanced hair loss. Hats and caps are many a woman's friend too. And no, wearing a hat does not cause hair loss (a common myth).

There are many solutions for instant cover-up which you can use every day while you work on the longer-term solutions.

MICRONUTRIENT DEFICIENCIES

You may have heard that taking certain vitamins or minerals as supplements can help slow or stop hair loss. This is only partly true.

If hair fall is due to, or associated with, a specific vitamin or mineral deficiency then replacing the nutrient in your diet, or using a supplement, is more likely to result in an improvement in hair quality and growth. If, however, your hair loss is not related to a nutrient deficiency, there is little to no evidence that supplements will help.

Below is a quick rundown of the most common vitamins and minerals that **may** have an impact on hair loss. I'd advise a visit to your doctor to discuss bloodwork to investigate your nutritional status, rather than taking guesses with supplements based on well-meaning but unqualified advice from other women.

Please do not increase your intake of any vitamin or mineral using a supplement without checking with your doctor first. While hair loss can be the result of a deficiency in some of these essential nutrients, there are significant side effects linked to taking too many.

IRON

A lot has been written about the connection between iron and hair loss[27], so you're probably not surprised to see it at the top of the list.

If low iron is causing your hair loss, you will probably notice a diffuse type of hair loss. This is a condition where more than normal amounts of hair are shed, resulting in an overall appearance of 'thinning hair'. Often the first thing a woman notices with this type of hair loss is the increased visibility of the scalp through the hair, or a much thinner ponytail.

Hair thinning of this nature can happen relatively quickly, but for some it can also happen very slowly, even over a period of years. Although it has been observed in all age groups, iron deficiency is the most common cause of hair loss in pre- and post-menopausal women.[28]

Iron is an essential mineral, required for numerous bodily functions and processes including immunity, synthesis of DNA, and the transmission of nerve signals. Iron is required for the creation of red blood cells and is also a major component of haemoglobin, the protein in the red blood cells that is responsible for carrying oxygen around in our blood. Iron is also an essential component of healthy hair.

You are probably familiar with fatigue as a key symptom of low or deficient iron. The mechanism for this is that the *serum iron,* that is the iron circulating in your blood stream, carries oxygen around the body. All cells need oxygen, so reduced function and exhaustion comes with inadequate oxygenation.

Stored iron is known as *ferritin.* When the serum iron drops, the body starts to call on its stored iron - its ferritin supplies. By the time a blood test shows low serum iron levels, the body will have exhausted its iron reserves. This is why it can take a long time to right any iron deficiency, replenish iron stores and restart the hair growth cycle.

However, low serum iron alone is not an indicator of an iron deficiency, it can also be an indication of other forms of chronic disease. For this reason and for your general health and wellbeing do not take iron supplements without medical supervision.

Specific to healthy hair, ferritin is needed in abundance by the hair follicles for optimal structure and function.

To find out if your iron levels are low, you will need to visit your doctor for a blood test. To test for low iron, they will likely order several different tests:

- serum iron (to see how much iron is circulating around your blood stream)
- ferritin (to gauge the amount of iron stores you have)
- transferrin (the main iron transporting protein)
- supplemental tests (including red cell count and haemoglobin levels that can suggest how well your body uses iron).

These will provide an overall picture of your iron levels and how well your body is using and storing iron, and offer a good starting point for investigation.

Low iron can result in hair loss because the body, when it is low in iron, uses less on non-essential processes such as maintaining and growing hair, thus leaving what is available for life-sustaining essentials like cellular oxygen supply.

When ferritin stores in the hair follicles decline, the hair that is produced will often be dry, brittle, non-pigmented and fine or thin. Because low iron stores deplete both the number of hairs on your head and their volume, it takes some time for the hair cycle to recover from an iron deficiency.

Iron is also important for optimal functioning of the immune system. Therefore, low iron can also lead to hair loss conditions like alopecia areata, which have an immunological involvement.

Please do not take iron supplements based on your reading here (or anywhere else). Too much iron can be dangerous and you should only take a supplement on the advice of your doctor based on investigations of your blood.

When should I suspect low iron?

Some of the most common symptoms associated with low iron levels include:

- general fatigue
- weakness
- pale skin
- shortness of breath
- dizziness
- brittle nails
- a tingling or 'crawling' feeling in the legs (restless legs)
- swelling or soreness in the tongue
- strange cravings for non-food items (such as dirt, ice or clay)
- cold hands and feet
- a fast or irregular heartbeat
- headaches
- changes in teeth and gums.

The only symptom of low iron I personally experienced, other than my hair loss and general fatigue, was my teeth. I made an appointment with my dentist because I noticed a few of my molars were loose. She checked my gums and said they were relatively healthy and intact; certainly not bad enough to cause my teeth to fall out. She asked me if my iron was low, and bingo! I said it was and as far as I knew at the time, had always been on the low side.

I thank God every day for that dentist. If she hadn't pointed to my dental issues being caused by low iron, I may not have sought to rectify the issue for many more months or even years.

If you are having any issues with your teeth and gums that are otherwise unexplained, have your iron checked. You only get one set of adult teeth.

Please consider also that many of the symptoms listed above can be attributed to other causes and factors. Because taking iron supplements when they are not needed can be very dangerous, always have your iron levels checked before taking it as a supplement.

What can I do about low iron?

If you are iron deficient, or your stores are low, your doctor will give you some recommendations, which may include iron supplements and diet changes.

Some foods that are rich in iron include:

- red meat, pork, poultry and seafood
- dark green leafy vegetables
- beans, legumes and pumpkin seeds
- some dried fruit such as raisins and apricots
- iron-fortified foods (e.g. cereals and breads).

Will my hair grow back if I am low in iron?

Yes, it definitely can. I am living proof.

Be patient though. It can take some time (even years) for hair to regrow after low iron levels, because your iron levels need to be restored first before the body can re-establish its focus on using that iron to grow healthy hair.

My own hair loss has gone through a range of causes and triggers over the years. I first experienced a brief spell of alopecia that quickly resolved (remember my patchy visit to the hairdresser?), and then there was the hormone imbalance caused by a medication, and surgical menopause. But underlying these and a few other trigger events, was my dangerously low iron stores.

Immediately after my doctor had confirmed this with comprehensive blood tests, I began taking supplements under her prescription and guidance. It was at least 18 months before I could see my hair was really starting to look normal again.

What I now know is that since my iron stores were always low, this was an underlying cause and contributing factor to the other hair loss triggers. Ten years on, I still take iron supplements, while having regular checks to ensure my iron levels are at a safe level. My body seems to have difficulty storing and using iron, but I stay on top of my bloodwork to make sure I'm not overdoing it as part of my ongoing health maintenance.

If clinically diagnosed low iron is your problem, there is hope.

What if my iron is 'within normal limits'? Should I still supplement?

I talk to hundreds of women whose blood tests show that their iron is 'within normal limits'. That is, there is no clear deficiency shown. I sense the frustration in women who complain that their doctor has dismissed their hair loss concerns, simply because their iron levels are within the 'normal' range.

Please consider that there are multiple reasons for your hair loss as there are multiple reasons your iron could be low. Your ferritin levels, transferrin and serum iron all must be taken into consideration. As too, your general health and wellbeing.

You will need to trust your medical professional who may be considering more than your iron levels as they relate to your hair health.

If you are at the low end of the normal range, ask your doctor to consider whether this lower result may not be optimal for you. Specifically, it may not be optimal for hair growth 'for you'. Enquire if there are records of previous blood tests you have had and check if your iron has dropped or fluctuated over time.

According to *Tosti et al,*[29] *"North American and UK experts in the hair field believe that treatment for hair loss is enhanced when patients maintain a serum ferritin concentration greater than 70 ng/ml."* Although in that study the experts recommend iron supplementation when ferritin levels are below 30ng/ml.

Because I've been getting my iron tested regularly for over a decade, I've had the opportunity to look back through my results and see a pattern. I've been able to identify what is low 'for me' and have needed to effectively triple my iron levels, from just below the normal range to well within the normal range, to effect positive change in my hair growth. But at all times, I have done this in consultation with my doctor.

If you are still not convinced or happy with your doctor's reaction to your blood test results, then I would advise seeking a second opinion, rather than self-supplementing with iron.

VITAMIN D

Low vitamin D levels are extremely common, especially if you're someone who doesn't spend much time in the sun. In fact, in Australia one in every four people has a clinical vitamin D deficiency according to the Australian Bureau of Statistics.[30]

Vitamin D is an important nutrient for hair-cycle health, so it is certainly possible that correcting vitamin D deficiency could improve hair-loss symptoms. Interestingly, having low vitamin D can also affect your ability to store iron, compounding nutritional matters. If a blood test shows that your serum vitamin D is below the normal range (or even at the low end of the normal range) please discuss taking a supplement with your physician. I personally know many women who have improved their hair growth by getting their serum vitamin D levels into a healthy range.

ZINC

It's quite common to be low in zinc, especially if you sweat a lot. Sweat is one of the primary ways we lose zinc, and loss will be compounded if your diet does not include sufficient sources of this mineral.

Zinc is required in many essential bodily functions, including cell reproduction and maintenance of hormone levels, which can affect hair growth and cycles. Importantly, zinc plays a critical role in helping you to absorb other vitamins and minerals, so a lack of zinc can increase the likelihood of other deficiencies. A zinc deficiency is also easy to diagnose via a blood test, and easy to fix with supplements and diet changes.

B-COMPLEX VITAMINS

B-complex vitamins and hair growth (particularly biotin, which I detail later) often crop up as the topic *de jour* for hair loss bloggers. B vitamins, in fact, do play an important role in nervous system function, hormone regulation and in optimal immune system processes.

Many hair loss sufferers swear by B vitamins, usually recommended as a complex supplement with a particularly high biotin dose. They believe that they have not only grown more hair, but that their hair shafts are thicker and stronger as a result of taking them. I suspect this is likely due to a placebo effect since, as you will see later in the section on biotin, it is unlikely that someone is deficient in biotin to the extent that taking a supplement alone, reverses their hair loss.

While supplementing with B vitamins is considered fairly safe, and since vitamin B12 is vital for optimal brain function, this is a good vitamin to take regularly as you age. But again I stress, do not take large amounts of these or any other vitamins unless you have discussed this with your doctor.

HAIR LOSS SUPPLEMENT FORMULAS

If you are experiencing an unusual amount of hair loss, one of the first suggestions you may get from helpful friends is to 'check your vitamins'. It's a common belief that certain nutrients can help slow or stop hair loss altogether. But this is only partly true since it only relates to some of us: when we have a deficiency.

The truth is that most of us who eat a balanced diet get enough vitamins and minerals through our food. If you are concerned that a deficiency may be the cause of your hair loss, the first step should be a consult and blood test with your doctor, and not just popping a hair growth supplement or gummy to 'see what happens'. There are many companies preying on women's insecurities around wrinkles, weight, cellulite, exercise and now, hair loss. So it is not surprising that off-the-shelf supplements and gummies, in their bright and attractive packages, have been designed to beckon to us. And we respond with 'It can't hurt, but it might help'.

Hair loss in women is a complex problem, much more complex than it is for men. Early intervention in female hair loss can halt it, reverse it, or slow it down. So, putting off seeing a doctor doesn't make good sense. Whether you are fearful of a diagnosis, or embarrassed by your hair loss, a medical professional is still the best place to start.

There is a great deal of misinformation about vitamins and minerals pervading online hair loss forums. They are often spoken about as 'natural' and 'harmless'. If we stop and investigate the issues at hand, we may find they could, indeed, hurt – and not help one bit. Remember, too, that over-supplementing with nutrients you don't need can cause all kinds of problems, including hair loss!

The supplement aisle at supermarkets and pharmacies seems to be getting bigger and bigger. It can be overwhelming to navigate all the formulations available, and you're not alone in wondering where on earth to begin. But what is in hair growth supplements, especially the popular new 'gummy' formulations? What do they claim to do and what do they actually do?

No matter the brand, hair-growth supplements and gummies usually contain a mixture of vitamins and minerals with established biological functions in hair, skin, and nail health, sometimes in very high doses. Vitamins A, C, E, iron, selenium, vitamin D and biotin often feature, alongside filler ingredients, like rice flour and sugar, to turn the concoction of nutrients into something yummy and chewy: a gummy!

Hair-growth tablets, gummies and supplements are classed as dietary supplements, and as such regulating bodies class them as foods, not drugs or medicines.

Just soak that up for a minute.

It means that the hair-growth pills you may be buying online or at the supermarket are officially considered a food, not a remedy that contains a therapeutic amount of anything useful. If it did, it would be classed as a medicine.

Biotin is a buzzword vitamin with some drastic claims about reversing and improving hair loss. However, a review of published literature on the subject of biotin use for hair loss concludes 'Though its use as a hair and nail growth supplement is prevalent, research demonstrating the efficacy of biotin is limited'.[31]

It is true that biotin plays an important role in hair health, but most adults are getting enough in their daily diet and will not benefit from taking a supplement – they are not deficient. The recommended daily intake of biotin is 30 mcg; however one of the more popular hair growth supplements contains 5,000 mcg – 166 times the adult daily requirement. When taken twice a day as recommended, this equates to 330 times more than you need!

Excess biotin can affect the body's ability to absorb zinc and vitamin B5 and can negatively impact laboratory testing accuracy, especially when measuring thyroid and cardiac functions.[32]

This could ultimately lead to a misdiagnosis. The biotin issue illustrates how important it is to work in partnership with your medical practitioner when considering or taking supplements of any kind.

What do scientists say about hair supplements?

The lack of data on supplements and gummies for hair loss raises some red flags. In fact, a significant proportion of the studies conducted on hair growth supplements have been funded by the brands themselves, with no independent, third-party trials or research.

One of the most important things for you to understand is that **the supplement market is not universally regulated or standardised.**

In Australia the Therapeutic Goods Administration (TGA) monitors the claims made on supplement labels and therefore we often see very carefully worded claims such as 'may support healthy hair growth'. But note that this is because there is not likely to be any evidence to support the claim, only a possible link at best. So while the TGA is monitoring the claims made on products manufactured in Australia, they are not monitoring the labels of products that Australians can buy online, originating from elsewhere in the world.

According to the website of the Food and Drug Administration (FDA) in the USA, they do not have the authority to review dietary supplement products for safety and effectiveness before they are marketed.[33] Therefore, **manufacturers do not need to provide any proof of safety, efficacy, or quality prior to sale**. The responsibility lies entirely with the brand producing the supplement. I don't know about you, but alarm bells are ringing for me. If there is no standard for what a hair growth supplement must contain to be effective, can we be sure that any one of the many formulations available will have any effect?

Hair supplements, gummies and other products are increasingly popular the world over. Approximately half of the USA adult population reports using dietary supplements and, in most instances, they have self-prescribed.[34]

The global beauty supplement market was valued at $3.5 billion in 2016 and is projected to grow to $6.8 billion by the end of 2024.[35]

In short, we're spending bucketloads on products that are potentially unregulated, may be ineffective and totally unnecessary, or even problematic and dangerous.

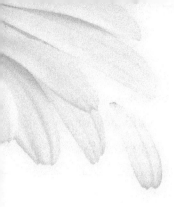

THE SCALP

Much like our garden needs great soil to grow healthy plants, so too our hair needs a well moisturised and healthy scalp to maintain healthy hair follicles.

To grow healthy hair, we need a healthy scalp.

FOLLICLES

Hair follicles are found just under the skin's surface all over the body, with the exception of the palms and soles of the feet. Hair follicles are made up of three essential structures:

- the dermal papilla
- the hair matrix
- the hair shaft.

The *matrix* surrounds the *papilla* and is responsible for producing the keratin protein that makes up the 'bulk' of the hair fibre. The matrix is also responsible for providing the melanin to give the hair its colour. Without the matrix, our hair would be transparent.

The *papilla* is found right at the base of the follicle, and perhaps has the most important role in gathering and storing nutrients from the blood vessels to 'feed' the follicle. When there are not enough nutrients in the circulating blood for the papilla to extract, this process breaks down.

While we know that the speed and pattern of hair growth is generally dependent on genetics, age, gender and hormones, we also know that nutritional deficiencies and hormone fluctuations can have a negative effect on healthy hair. It's not surprising, then, that a diet high in processed and fast foods, and lacking essential nutrients, may have a negative effect on our hair growth and its quality.

Whenever I'm asked why I believe female hair loss is more prevalent today than it was 60+ years ago, my answer is always that diet is one of the most obvious factors. The past decades have seen a change in our overall diets from more natural, whole foods to processed and fast foods, which usually deeply lack nutritional value.

SCALP HEALTH

We need healthy follicles to produce healthy hair – and healthy follicles require a healthy scalp, with good nutrition playing a major role. Quality hair care products that care for and nourish the scalp are also critical.

Like all skin on the body, our scalp is made up of three major 'layers':

- the dermis
- the epidermis
- the subcutaneous tissue.

While much has been written about hair follicles and their role in producing healthy hair, maintaining healthy cycles and hair shaft thickness, we must not neglect the skin that houses the follicle.

Many studies have been carried out on hair transplants and there are a plethora of papers and research on the subject.[36] One crucial factor in a successful hair transplant is the quality of the scalp tissue into which it is transplanted. It is clear that a healthy, intact hair follicle is needed for the survival of the hair transplant. These studies have shown that even with a healthy follicle, if the scalp skin is damaged or unhealthy, the follicle will struggle to produce and support healthy hair. This can result in thin and very fine hair shafts and a poor result.

There are many types of scalp health issues – some you can manage yourself while others will need investigation and support from a dermatologist.

One entirely preventable scalp health issue is excessive sun exposure. Just like the rest of our body, the scalp can become sunburnt very quickly and easily. If you have thinning hair your scalp is even more exposed and vulnerable to sun damage. It is not easy to put sunscreen on our head, so we tend not to think of it. Using a cotton bud to apply sunscreen to thin areas or the part line is one way to ensure you are not exacerbating a widening part with excessive sun exposure and resulting damage. Wearing a hat is the most efficient sun protection solution. While some people fear that wearing a hat could cause rubbing or friction that increases hair loss, that's a complete myth. A good hat will protect your scalp and hair.

For women with longer hair, wear a bun or ponytail to provide some protection, brushing the hair over your scalp.

Protecting your scalp from the damaging ultraviolet (UV) rays of the sun is an absolute must if you want to maintain optimal hair growth.

Hair fibres, preferably made from cotton, offer another way to hide your scalp from the sun. While they do not contain specific sun blocking properties like SPF, they may help to protect the scalp from exposure to the sun by acting as a physical barrier.

AGEING SKIN

All skin loses its elasticity with age. It also loses density and 'thins' as we get older. Our scalp undergoes the same changes. While our follicles reduce in size with age, thus producing a thinner hair shaft, our scalp skin ages along with it. So our hair, too, will show signs of age. While there are some signs of age-related hair loss we cannot do anything about, we can at least do everything we can to look after the skin on our scalp.

Often, the first noticeable symptom of ageing hair for a woman is a reduction in hair shaft thickness. For women with thick, dark-coloured hair, a thinner hair shaft may give the overall appearance of hair loss, when in fact it is simply that age has resulted in a thinner hair shaft, giving the overall appearance of less hair. These women may think they are losing hair, but each shaft is simply 'thinning'.

It makes perfect sense to us that a good quality facial cream with premium ingredients will help preserve and protect the skin on the face. We need to start considering our scalps with the same tender respect.

As a teenager I was taught that I should never condition the roots of my hair; that conditioner should be applied to the ends of the hair only. In fact, I recently read that conditioner should only be applied from the ears down – all very well, if your hair grows that long.

As we age, this advice is no longer relevant. If you are someone with very oily skin and oily hair, then this advice may not be for you. But for those with dry skin and hair, you may need to change the way you treat your scalp and hair in order to preserve hair quality, and hopefully its density, for as long as possible.

Conditioning technique

Firstly, apply conditioner gently into all parts of your hair – not just the ends – and apply it liberally to your scalp on a regular basis. Massaging the conditioner into your scalp can be beneficial for the massage as well as the moisture.

At least once a week, I suggest you use a hair mask before washing your hair. Take a good amount of the mask and apply it throughout your hair from root to tip. Wrap your hair in a hair towel or turban wrap, or loosely tie it up out of the way and leave the mask in for a good 10 minutes. Then wash and condition as usual.

This technique can be beneficial for dry and damaged hair and for ageing hair that is frizzy and unmanageable. I have been doing this for a long while now and the benefits are clearly visible.

You should also consider a lightweight, moisturising, leave-in spray that is kind to hair and contains nourishing ingredients. This will add moisture to dry hair and scalp between washes and treatments, and keep your hair moisturised.

The good news about increasing the moisture on your scalp (and therefore your hair) is that if your hair loss is exacerbated by poor quality hair strands, the repair masks and moisture sprays can improve scalp health and hair quality over the long term.

Boost & Be has a great range of shampoos, conditioners, masks and styling products that have been formulated especially for scalp and hair health. They contain none of the nasty chemicals that can further exacerbate hair loss or an unhealthy scalp environment.

SCALP PROBLEMS

Dozens of diseases can affect the scalp, from acne to dandruff, psoriasis to impetigo, herpes to melanoma. Other conditions that can affect the scalp include cradle cap, lupus and ringworm.

I would strongly suggest you see your doctor for a referral to a dermatologist if you suspect you have any of these problems. I have observed women with what appear to be very minor irritations of the scalp quickly develop significant hair loss, only to see them a year later and their hair growth has returned to normal again after treatment with a specialist.

DANDRUFF

Do you know that those troublesome flakes you brush off your shoulders may not be dandruff?

It's far more likely that they are caused by a dry scalp, which is not true dandruff. If you've wrongly 'diagnosed' yourself as a dandruff sufferer, specialty shampoos for this condition may end up making your condition worse.

What is dandruff?

Contrary to popular belief, dandruff is not caused by scalp dryness. Rather, true dandruff results from an excess of sebum – natural skin oils that accumulate on the scalp and lead to an overgrowth of yeasts and fungi – not scalp dryness. These factors can cause skin cells to shed more frequently, giving you that 'fresh from a snowstorm' look. Unlike dry scalp though, true dandruff has a yellowish tint and is greasy rather than dry and flaky.

Like many hair and skin issues dandruff can be caused by a number of factors. There may be a physical cause such as poor nutrition (especially a diet too high in fat, sugars and/ or starches), hormones, heredity or scalp sensitivity. Dandruff can also be a by-product of stress, of being generally run down, or of infrequent hair washing, or misuse or excessive use of styling products.

Treatment

Anti-dandruff shampoos take up a lot of space on the market. They include some strong, medicated ingredients in their formulations, designed to treat the inflammation and yeast build-up on your scalp. But these same ingredients can also exacerbate and irritate a dry scalp. Make sure you're dealing with true dandruff before using dandruff products, or your issue may worsen.

A lot of people mistakenly believe that it is best to avoid frequent shampooing when dandruff is present; however, the opposite is true. You need to keep the excess oil at bay, so that yeast and fungi cannot proliferate. Washing every second day should be sufficient, but if you're noticing that your scalp remains excessively oily, wash it every day with a specialty shampoo until the problem is under control.

Dry scalp

Dry skin can occur anywhere on the body, including the scalp. Chronic scalp dryness is likely to be an itchy condition and the flakes are smaller, whiter, and more brittle than true dandruff flakes. Scalp 'burn' due to a lack of sun protection is one of the leading causes of a dry scalp – often mistaken, and subsequently mistreated, as dandruff.

Let's return to our garden analogy – I think of a dry scalp much like the cracked, dry and parched earth we see during a drought. We know that nothing can grow and thrive there. Similarly, a dry scalp, lacking in natural oils and moisture, will struggle to keep hair follicles healthy and to nurture healthy hair growth.

If your visible flakes are the result of a dry scalp, there's a lot you can do and it pays dividends to get it under control. A concerted effort to change your hair management regimen is required, building in the following steps:

- using conditioner from root to tip
- massaging an oil or repair mask into your scalp as part of your regular conditioning treatment (and occasionally overnight)
- protecting your scalp from the sun (using sunscreen and/or a hat).

Scalp care takes some effort, but it yields thicker, more manageable hair and solves the embarrassing 'snowstorm' problem.

SMOKING

Did you know that smoking is bad for your hair? Specifically, it's your hair follicles that pay the price.

An observational study carried out in Switzerland in 2003 confirmed a significant link between tobacco smoking and baldness.[37] It had previously been thought that cigarette smoke caused damage to the DNA of the hair follicle, thus impeding its natural growth cycle. However, this study found that the mechanism appears to relate to the effects of the smoke itself on the dermal papilla of the follicle, rather than nicotine and/ or other chemicals and additives taken into the body.

None of this should be surprising since we are familiar with the damage smoking does to the skin, causing premature ageing and early greying of the hair.

If you needed new motivation to create a quit plan and finally give up cigarettes, then perhaps this is the message you need to hear.

STRESS

Stress is a silent killer. It affects our wellbeing at every level.

I've already touched on stress as a huge factor in FPHL but let's take a deeper dive. Stress is a common and often overlooked cause of hair loss in women. Recall that the type of hair loss caused by acute stress it is known as telogen effluvium.

When you picture stress-induced hair loss, you might be thinking of someone quite literally tearing their hair out, running around trying to get their life together. Stress and overwhelm can, in fact, trigger hair loss on their own – no pulling required!

You may remember the concept of 'fight or flight' from high school biology. It describes how, when in sudden and present danger, our brain launches a hormonal response to the threat.

This in turn raises our blood pressure causing faster breathing and an expansion of the airways in our lungs, dilating our blood vessels and releasing glucose into our blood stream. There is an increase in the flow of oxygen and fuel around the body in tandem with these responses, especially to the muscles. With this burst of energy, we can respond effectively to the threat.

But in these modern times we're less exposed to immediate threats and are more vulnerable to long-term, low-level chronic stress. Constant worry about a loved one, financial stressors, an abusive or difficult relationship or, in more recent times, the fear and stresses associated with living through a pandemic, are interpreted by our body as threats to survival, with similarly intense biological responses.

High levels of continued stress are particularly difficult for our bodies to cope with. We are forced to constantly adjust, which is a stressor itself and can lead to the development of chronic diseases. High blood pressure, heart disease, obesity, diabetes, and inflammatory conditions (such as Crohn's disease and arthritis) all have strong correlations with chronic stress.

There is also mounting evidence that stress affects our brain function, causing memory loss and cognitive decline. The inflammatory repercussions of stress have been linked to dementia and Alzheimer's disease specifically, showing us that stress, brain function and inflammation are all interconnected. Similarly, we know that chronic inflammation can lead to the suppression of immune system function, which can lead to diseases like cancer and some autoimmune conditions.

Many of us with hair loss also understand firsthand that stress plays a huge role in the development and severity of our condition. The mechanisms involved in stress and hair loss have been the subject of many scientific studies, confirming our experiences.

A pilot study on young, healthy women, conducted in Germany in 2017 by the National Centre for Biotechnology indicated that stress during a high-tension exam period can cause an interruption to the natural hair growth cycle.[38] Another study concluded that: 'stress has long been implicated as one of the causal factors involved in hair loss' and that even stress caused by experiencing hair loss is a significant contributing factor to hair loss itself.[39] Take note ladies – it can truly be a vicious cycle.

The suggestion 'don't stress about your hair loss' is much easier said than done. However, I do firmly believe in actively moderating and managing your stress about it to the best of your capacity: recall my first experience with hair loss with my hairdresser pointing out a patch of alopecia areata. I completely forgot about it and within a few months it was completely gone. My ignorance at that time may have served me well.

Since I began using cotton hair fibres, I don't stress about my hair loss being noticed, as I am perfectly camouflaging it. This provides significant relief from stress for me and its effect on my self-esteem.

A word to the wise: if you are someone who is counting, collecting and even bagging up your shed hair (many women do this – I've seen the social media posts). please stop this practice. It can contribute enormously to your stress levels. If you are collecting shed hair, then you most probably have TE, and you know now that this will resolve. Give it time. Look after your general health and your hair health, and know that you are doing all you can to give your body what it needs to recover. Managing your stress is critical for all aspects of health.

It is next to impossible to avoid stress altogether in the 21st century, but you can take steps to reduce it in your life and carve out time and space that nourishes you over the long term.

The stressors I've covered so far are obvious and we feel the frustration of these life events clearly. We know our bodies are not coping due to the lack of good sleep or feelings of anger and frustration bubbling up.

But there is a source of stress that most of us are not inherently aware of: a compounding of lifestyle factors that can wreak havoc over time.

Many women are doing too much, often with the combination of a high stress work environment, along with the lions share of responsibility for childbearing and raising children or caring for extended family and ageing parents. The combination of full-time work, juggling a family, poor dietary choices and being constantly time-poor with no 'down time' has resulted in increasingly younger women presenting with chronic weight gain, heart disease, hair loss and other chronic illnesses.

Compounded stress also leads to a sustained increase in specific stress hormones, like cortisol. When these hormones are elevated long term, it can damage blood vessels, increasing the likelihood of developing high blood pressure, heart attacks and strokes.

Chronically elevated stress hormones also alter the body's use of energy stores. Appetite can increase, leading to the build-up of fat stores and weight gain, which can, in turn, lead to further systemic inflammation.

Ultimately, inflammation is why stress is known as the 'silent killer' and is a major contributing cause of female hair loss. So, what can we do about it?

Following are answers to some of the questions I get asked most frequently about stress and hair loss for women.

HOW DOES STRESS CAUSE HAIR LOSS?

Understanding the hair growth cycle is the key to under-standing why stress can cause hair loss, which is covered in detail in an earlier chapter. You will recall that hair growth is cyclical, passing through three main stages: the growth phase (anagen), the resting phase (catagen) and finally, the shedding phase (telogen).

Under normal circumstances we have an average of 100,000 hairs on our head and shed a small percentage of these on a daily basis as a healthy process. When something disrupts the hair growth cycle, like stress, the cycle can be interrupted. This could result in more hairs entering the shedding stage at one time, or follicles may not grow a new hair once a hair is shed.

This occurs because growing hair isn't a priority for the body when it is under stress – lustrous hair is a bonus, not a survival necessity. If you're stressed, your body focuses on just keeping your most essential processes and functions going and neglects 'unimportant' tasks, like keeping your hair healthy and plentiful.

WHAT CONSTITUTES STRESS?

Stress is a very broad term, especially when it comes to hair loss. It certainly refers to **emotional** stress, but it also refers to **physical** stress, such as gaining or losing a significant amount of weight, going through surgery or coping with illness. We may not consider physical factors as stressful but our bodies certainly do.

When we talk about physical stress we are not talking about exercise. A busy life, regular gym workouts, a physical job, running around after children all day, lifting, carrying, cycling, climbing, sports and generally 'sweating it out' are all good and healthy activities and don't constitute physical stress. In fact, physical fitness is extremely beneficial for reducing overall stress and maintaining health. Physical stressors can be illnesses, accidents, infections, surgeries and shocks, and the severity and type of the physical stress required to trigger hair loss will vary from person to person. While some will not experience hair loss even after getting through a life-threatening illness, others could lose hair after a swift bout of gastroenteritis.

Regarding emotional stress, it is unlikely that you will experience hair loss due to acute low levels of stress, like being late for work or forgetting an important appointment. But the death of a loved one or a complicated divorce, or even moving house can be particularly unsettling and may affect your hair cycles.

Still, everyday stressors can have other negative health effects, so if you feel stressed often, it's a good idea to discuss this with your GP.

HOW LONG DOES HAIR TAKE TO RECOVER AFTER STRESS?

Hair loss caused by stress usually only becomes evident several months after the onset of the stress. Therefore it will take several months for the hair cycle to restabilise after a period of intense stress has resolved. Once the hair cycle has normalised, it will take further time to regrow and 'fill in' sparse areas of the scalp.

The short answer is: at least 6 to 12 months after your stress is resolved.

Note also that if your hair doesn't seem to be recovering from TE, then there is likely to be something else at play. There could be one or more of the underlying causes I've mentioned preventing your body from recovering from TE.

HOW CAN I PREVENT LOSING HAIR DUE TO STRESS?

Stress on its own doesn't cause hair loss in every woman. While stress is the **trigger** that causes the hair loss, it is the presence of one or more **underlying causes** that allows the trigger to have an effect.

To prevent any future bouts of TE or stress-related hair loss, paying attention to your overall health, and your hair health in particular, is key.

If you find yourself in a constant state of stress, which can have other debilitating effects on your overall health, then the best first action is to visit your GP. They may be able to refer you to a good counsellor or psychologist who can assist you to identify stressors in your life and to find ways to cope with or minimise them. A doctor can also order blood tests and other investigations to ensure that there is no underlying medical condition or deficiency that may be contributing to your stress and, therefore, your hair loss.

Improvements to your diet, your sleep quality and your stress levels are tightly interconnected, and it is much easier said than done to address these.

While there are many websites, books and gurus providing advice on each of these three key factors, I believe in one thing that can have a huge healing effect on our body, mind and soul, attending to all three at once: breathing.

Breathing

I have been purposefully using breathing techniques for many years now. I know this may sound like crazy talk if you haven't encountered it before. But a quick Google search will yield thousands of pages on breathing and health. You don't need to practice meditation or yoga to breathe well. Anyone can do it.

I initially began using breathing techniques to improve my memory. I was aware that my memory was being affected due to my body's response to stress (elevated cortisol, insulin resistance and chronic inflammation) and I felt I wasn't at my sharpest.

I did a great deal of research on memory improvement techniques and I tried them all. I love a good cryptic crossword and started doing more of those with the intention of boosting my overall brain function. While this may well have proven to be a good strategy, I found that I really didn't have the time to sit and nut out a cryptic puzzle each and every day.

My research led me to the work of neuroscientist, Professor Ian Robertson, and his message that deliberate, deep breathing is the brain's 'reset button' and the most precise, accessible and side-effect-free 'pharmaceutical' that could ever be prescribed.[40]

Breathing exercises are known to reduce stress levels, improve memory and cognitive function, as well as help you ease back to sleep if you wake.[41] [42]

Applying breathing techniques frequently makes a considerable difference to your energy levels and can help you moderate and control your stress responses. When practised regularly, over time, breathing techniques help to set your body's default at a calmer and more stable resting state. This has the potential to reduce chronic inflammation, helping to resolve or improve a host of conditions, and subsequently, assisting the health of your hair to improve.

Breathing techniques do form the backbone of meditation, yoga and tai chi, so if you are interested in learning more of these embodiment arts then they can definitely improve your overall health.

Here are some simple, quick exercises you can adopt into your daily life to get you started and quickly bring vast improvements.

The '4–7–8' breath
Breathe in through your nose for the count of 4, hold for a count of 7 and exhale through your mouth to the count of 8. You can do this any time – in a meeting, during the night when you are lying awake, during the day when you notice your breathing is shallow or that you are having trouble concentrating. Or if,

like me, you have a smart watch, you may use a setting that reminds you to breathe mindfully at regular intervals through the day. Complete up to 10 cycles of this breath or continue it for as long as it feels right for you. It may take a while to get used to, and you may find yourself yawning the first few times you try this. But with practice, your body will adjust and it will simply feel good and energising.

Repeat a couple of times a day, or whenever you think of it.

Alternate nostril breathing (ANB)

This is a traditional breathing exercise used in the yoga tradition and has many documented benefits, specifically for the brain. In ANB, you block one nostril with the index finger, breathe in through the other nostril for 5 seconds, hold for 5, then block the nostril you just breathed in with and breathe out through the other nostril. Alternate between nostrils for 5 full cycles, beginning and ending on the left nostril. As you practice this exercise over time, you may find that you can increase the cycles with even more benefit.

The simple art of breathing can have a positive effect on your mind, your body, your stress levels and ultimately, your hair.

HOW CAN I HELP MY HAIR GROW BACK AFTER STRESS?

Hair loss caused by acute stress will usually right itself in time: you will have to let the shedding run its course. I know that can feel disheartening if you are in the middle of a massive shed. I think every woman who has been through it will sympathise with you (and they frequently do in online support groups).

Take time to do some nice things for yourself. Get your nails done, have a pedicure, a massage, go for a long swim, arrange a date night with your significant other or make more effort to catch up for coffee or go to a movie with friends.

Divert your thinking and attention away from your hair loss towards enjoyable and inspiring topics and activities.

Remember the stress of worrying about hair loss causes more hair loss.

Use cover-up techniques like cotton hair fibres to give you added confidence when you are out and about. Their camouflage effect offers great relief.

Patience is the key to working with your body to grow your hair back. Commit to healthy hair habits and healthy hair products.

Above all, be kind to yourself.

Hair pulling (trichotillomania)

Trichotillomania is an impulse control disorder where the sufferer has an overwhelming urge to pull their hair out. They may pull out head hair, eyebrows, eyelashes, beard hair or any other hair covering their body, often until they are visibly balding.

Doctors are unclear about the causes of trichotillomania. Some studies have focused on it as a form of addiction or obsessive tendency, while others have focused on a correlation with mental health conditions, such as anxiety and depression.[43]

Many trichotillomania patients show improvement with psychotherapy and hypnosis techniques; however, there is no known guaranteed cure.

If you think you may have trichotillomania, please visit your doctor. You may be given a referral to a psychologist or other specialist who can help you get to the bottom of why you are pulling your hair. There are also some great organisations that provide support and advice to people with trichotillomania. A quick search on the internet should bring up an organisation close to you, or you may find some online support services.

HAIR CARE PRACTICES

Hair loss isn't always caused by a physiological change. It could be that you are mistreating or mishandling your hair without even knowing it in your care regime, leading to breakage and poor hair quality. Here's where hair care techniques, products and knowledge are important.

HEATED STYLING

Hair dryers, hot rollers, curling wands and hair straighteners are notorious for causing hair breakage. The excessive heat required to change the shape of your hair dries and 'fries' it at the same time.

If you must use heated styling equipment, nurture your hair with a high quality conditioner and use a leave-in moisturiser. Consider the regular use of a heat protection spray before styling and choose equipment that has variable heat settings so you can control the level of heat directly affecting your hair.

PERMING AND STRAIGHTENING

Do you know every aspect of your hairdresser's life back to front? If so, you may be visiting a little too often.

Most of us are aware that the chemical preparations used by hairdressers to alter the look of our hair are not ideal for the overall quality and health of our hair. Perming and straightening solutions have certainly improved over the years and don't 'cook' our hair like they did in the '80s. However, they do still dry the hair and cause it to become more brittle, leading to hair breakage and loss.

If you really can't live without perming or straightening, consider investing in an intensive hair treatment each time you go to the salon.

TIGHT, PULLED BACK HAIRSTYLES

Wearing your hair in a tight ponytail, a bun or in tight braids every day can cause a type of alopecia called *traction alopecia* which occurs around the front of the hair line. The constant pulling on the hair follicle initially causes inflammation of the follicle. The first sign that something is wrong is often visible bumps and redness which appear around the follicle. If left untreated the hair follicle will scar and stop growing altogether. This is known as scarring alopecia. It is common in women of colour and women who wear tight braids, weaves and wigs.

If you continue to put your hair under this kind of tension long term, the damage can be permanent. The good news is that if you give your hair a break from this kind of stress, the follicles can recover.

One way to relieve your follicles from this stress is to ask your hair stylist to apply your pulled back style a little more gently and a little looser.

HAIRSPRAYS, MOUSSES AND GELS

Loading up on styling products to get your look just right may be the only way to manage your thinning hair. But while light use of your favourite products is reasonable, going overboard may dehydrate and weaken hair.

Steer clear of heavy gels that cause your hair to become super sticky; instead opt for lighter, moisturising hair sprays – they style just as well. Further, avoid brushing out styling products as this is likely to cause a lot of hair breakage. Instead, gently rinse out your products with water before you shampoo. Use gentle, kind-to-hair shampoos and conditioners. If tangles remain, use a wide-toothed comb to apply conditioner throughout the hair. This will minimise the damage and breakage from trying to brush knots out of dry, brittle hair.

HAIR DYE

Do hair dyes cause hair loss?

This is one of the most frequent questions I field from women, and there is no simple answer. Rather, the 'answer' is: no … probably not … but maybe.

When we dye our hair, we are essentially applying chemicals to something that is dead. Once the hair has reached the skin's surface, it no longer contains any living cells. Hair grows from the follicle at the root, which is nourished via the bloodstream. It is for this reason that many people assume that hair dyes couldn't possibly cause hair loss. For the most part, that is true. However, there are some rare instances where hair dye **may** be the cause of, or at least a contributing factor to, hair loss.

In some people, certain hair dyes can penetrate the hair follicle itself, causing it to die or become inactive. It is not known why this happens for some people and not others, but some experts speculate that an allergy or reaction to certain chemicals may be implicated.[44] This may relate to individual hair, skin and follicle types. It is important to note that dyeing hair is extremely unlikely to be the reason for your hair loss but there are some factors regarding hair dyeing that are worthy of discussion.

Firstly, it is possible that your hair may appear thinner if you are regularly colouring it. If you are lightening your hair, this involves stripping out some of the pigment and nutrient from the surface of the hair shaft, making your hair potentially finer, drier and more brittle. Brittle and dry hair tends to break more easily, leading to the appearance of hair loss. Additionally, lighter hair tends to look less dense and the scalp will show through more readily under very light hair. If you have decided to lighten your hair as you age, then you may be noticing visibly thinner hair, which is not necessarily hair loss but the simple phenomenon that lighter hair is actually finer. If you are darkening your hair, then you are adding pigment to a hair shaft that otherwise is lacking it. Hair dyed darker can tend to look denser and hence thicker.

I have continued to dye my hair throughout my hair loss years. Given that I have grown my hair back while still dyeing it every three to four weeks, I can definitely conclude it has had no effect on my personal hair health at all.

Bear in mind that while darker hair may look thicker, it could make thinning hair more visibly noticeable for an entirely different reason. Dark hair is a vastly different colour to a light scalp, particularly in fair-skinned individuals. The contrast between the hair and the scalp is thus more noticeable, especially if your hair is being lost in patches.

The visibility of the scalp through the hair is the number one embarrassing element reported by women suffering hair loss. This is why cotton hair fibre concealers, like Boost N Blend, have become so popular and work so well. Their primary purpose is to thicken each strand of hair to obscure the visibility of the scalp.

Cotton hair fibres come in a variety of colours. By simply shaking them onto dry hair you will add extra volume at the roots. The cotton fibres cling to the hair shaft, making it up to 10 times thicker. This extra volume at the roots eliminates the contrast between dark hair and a light scalp so that visible hair loss completely vanishes. For women with lighter coloured hair that is actually finer, also resulting in a visible scalp, lighter cotton hair fibres fill in the hair diameter, thus making the hair look thicker.

Minimising the impact of hair dyes

If you have undergone all the relevant blood tests and investigations, perhaps even seen a specialist, and have still not found a reason for your hair loss, then the only way to determine if hair dye is the culprit is to stop dyeing it for several months and see if your hair loss eases.

This strategy may be out of the question for many of you but there are some tips to minimise the impact of hair dye on hair loss.

Find a salon that uses natural dyes

When hair dyes cause, or affect, hair loss it is usually due to a specific chemical or combination of chemicals used in the dyeing product, rather than the dyeing itself. If you tend to be sensitive to chemicals or have sensitive skin, it's a good idea to stay away from harsh chemical hair products. There are a growing number of salons that use minimal chemicals in their colouring products, with staff trained to take extra care for women with hair loss.

Consider 'off-scalp' hair colouring

Foils, for example, are a good way to colour your hair without applying the product directly onto your scalp. Foils and tips can give the overall appearance of a fresh colour without the risk of scalp irritation or inflammation. Try highlighting to lighten hair all over, or lowlighting to darken the appearance of your hair.

Use natural and organic hair products

Slathering your scalp with chemical-laden shampoos, conditioners and styling products is completely unnecessary and can be harmful. See the section called Hair Care Products for tips on the healthiest selections.

Part III

How to minimise, prevent and disguise hair loss

SUPPLEMENTS

BIOTIN

If you've done your research about hair loss, you've no doubt heard about biotin – a so-called 'miracle' cure for hair loss.

The claims made about this nutrient are so prevalent that it could deserve its own chapter. Read on to potentially save yourself a lot of wasted hope, money and some horrible side effects.

Firstly, you must know that there are no scientific studies to suggest that someone with hair loss will see any improvement in their condition by consuming biotin supplements, particularly if they are not deficient in biotin.

Biotin deficiency is very rare and so it's highly unlikely to be the cause of your hair loss. Symptoms of biotin deficiency include dry scaly skin, cracking in the corners of the mouth, swollen and painful tongue, dry eyes, loss of appetite, fatigue, insomnia, and depression.

What is biotin?

Biotin is a B-complex vitamin, sometimes also referred to as 'Vitamin H'.

Like all B-group vitamins biotin is water soluble so your body doesn't store it. This has led many to assume that we need to be constantly replenishing our bodies with biotin supplements but this is simply not the case.

Biotin can be made in the intestine and is also found in a wide variety of foods; this is why biotin deficiencies are extremely rare.[45]

Biotin is found in dairy products, egg yolks, oily fish (such as sardines, salmon and tuna), nuts (pecans, almonds, peanuts, walnuts), soybeans, legumes (beans, black-eyed peas), chicken and liver. It is also prevalent in many fruits and vegetables including bananas, mushrooms and cauliflower, as well as in whole grains and brewer's yeast.

Anyone eating a healthy, varied diet is likely to have sufficient biotin in their system.

How much biotin do I need?

While it is true that biotin plays an important role in the health of your hair, most adults are getting enough biotin through their diet alone and will not benefit from taking a biotin supplement.

A non-breastfeeding adult only requires 30 mcg daily (35 mcg for those breastfeeding)[46] and many of the supplements found on the shelves range from 300 mcg to a whopping 10,000 mcg, with the most common dose being 5,000 mcg. Furthermore, many of these companies suggest taking one tablet twice a day!

A common source of confusion is the difference between a microgram (mcg) and a milligram (mg). They are not the same thing. One milligram (mg) is equal to 1000 micrograms (mcg). So if you are taking a supplement with 50 **mg** of biotin you are in serious trouble, because that is 50,000 **mcg.**

Many people believe it's perfectly safe to take a large amount of vitamin or mineral supplements, presumably because they are perceived as healthy and natural; however, without the supervision of your doctor, excessive supplements really can cause problems.

Can I have too much biotin?

Yes!

Biotin negatively interacts with the body's ability to absorb both zinc and vitamin B5 (pantothenic acid), meaning that excessive intake of biotin can cause a deficiency in one or both of these nutrients.

If you've been reading carefully you may remember that a potential side effect of a zinc deficiency is hair loss.

And guess what a potential side effect of a B5 deficiency is? Hair loss!

So, you will potentially risk worsening your hair loss by taking the massive amounts of biotin in many hair growth formulas. Even if you are biotin deficient, you certainly don't need thousands of micrograms per day.

Another common side effect of taking biotin (especially in high doses) is acne, which occurs due to the lowering of your B5 levels.

To summarise, biotin is probably not going to cure your hair loss and may actually make your hair loss worse and harm you in other ways.

Some interesting facts about biotin:

- Raw egg whites bind with biotin in the small intestine and prevent it from being absorbed. Eating two or more raw egg whites a day over several months can lead to a biotin deficiency.
- Alcohol is known to reduce the body's absorption of the B-group vitamins, including biotin.

PUMPKIN SEED OIL

There has been a lot of online discussion in women's hair loss groups and in the media around the use of pumpkin seed oil as a treatment for hair loss. As far as I can tell, this is all based on a study conducted in 2014 on 76 men [47] although there is another study published in 2019 which was conducted on mice [48].

In the 2014 study, the male participants were given a 400mg capsule to take once a day for 24 weeks. This capsule contained other ingredients including evening primrose powder, red clover powder, tomato powder and corn silk.

While a positive hair count increase was seen in all participants at the end of the trial, it could not be said that the results were due to the pumpkin seed oil alone, because it was used in conjunction with the other ingredients.

Pumpkin seed oil is known for its antiandrogenic effect on rats. And the men in this trial had mild to moderate androgenic alopecia which is the result of circulating male hormones being converted into DHT on the scalp.

Like so many of the treatments currently available, they have been developed by men, for men, and have been specifically developed or tested, to treat androgenic alopecia.

As I pointed out earlier, many scientists [49] now believe that women do not respond to antiandrogenic therapy in the same way as men, due to the fact that female hair loss is not caused by the same hormonal factors as men's hair loss.

VITAMIN A

A healthy hair follicle contains cells that are rapidly dividing. Like any bodily function it needs good nutritional support to operate at its optimum. For this reason, many women look to vitamins and over-the-counter supplements to boost the health of their hair.

Vitamin A is one such vitamin that has been linked to healthy hair. According to a review of vitamins and minerals in hair loss published in *Dermatology and Therapy*, [50] a balanced diet will supply a sufficient amount of vitamin A. It also notes that high levels of vitamin A can be toxic and can in fact, cause hair loss when taken in high doses.

Like all supplements, do not take them unless you have a diagnosed deficiency.

VITAMIN C

Vitamin C plays an important role in the body's ability to absorb iron. If you are taking iron for a diagnosed deficiency, then you may have been told to take your iron with vitamin C containing foods.

There is no specific data which correlates a lack of vitamin C with hair loss[51].

SELENIUM

While selenium is required by the body to grow healthy hair, it unlikely that someone with a normal diet would require supplementation. A healthy diet including meat, vegetables and nuts would contain sufficient selenium to meet daily requirements.

There was an outbreak of acute selenium poisoning in 2008 [52] which was traced back to a liquid dietary supplement that contained 200 times the labelled concentration of selenium. Of the 201 cases identified with selenium toxicity, hair loss was a reported symptom in 75% of the cases.

Other symptoms included diarrhoea, fatigue, joint pain, nail discolouration and brittleness and nausea.

There is another good reason not to take supplements that you may have heard someone mention in association with hair loss.

DIET AND NATURAL METHODS

You know the truth of the adage: *You are what you eat* – Right?

It isn't a huge leap to understand that the quality of those less-than-luscious locks you've been worried about may have something to do with what's passing through your mouth.

In fact, diet is one of the first areas you should improve to optimise hair, skin and nail health.

PROTEIN

Do you get enough protein from your diet?

Many women are not eating sufficient protein. Since your body needs protein to make hair strong, you may find that adding a protein powder to your daily regimen or increasing your general protein intake from other sources may help to keep your hair in healthier shape.

Meat, fish and eggs are great sources. If you are vegetarian be sure to include the minimum recommended amount of protein for your weight and activity level from legumes, nuts and other sources.

Did you know that some of the most common, and delicious, dietary proteins have additional beneficial effects for our hair?

- **Milk** is a primary source of calcium, which is needed for vitamin D absorption. Recent studies have uncovered a link between low vitamin D and hair loss in women.[53] Vitamin D has many other protective benefits too, so it may be worth having your levels checked if you think you could be lacking. Either way, you need good dietary sources and a burst of sunshine each day.
- **Eggs** are also a great source of vitamin D, as well as B-complex vitamins, which are involved in the development of keratin.
- **Salmon** is a significant source of biotin and has other important benefits as well. Oily fish like salmon contain omega-3 fatty acids, which are

vital for healthy, well-moisturised skin and, in turn, a healthy scalp.

IRON

Red meat is an excellent iron source, but if you're vegetarian or don't eat it for other reasons, there are lots of other ways to ensure a good dietary intake of this critical mineral.

Vegetarians may need to keep a closer eye on their iron levels, however, as the type of iron found in plants is not as readily absorbed as the type of iron found in meats. Try to eat more green leafy vegetables, legumes (especially white beans and lentils) and quinoa. Remember that vitamin C helps to absorb iron, so eating foods rich in vitamin C with foods rich in iron is a great idea. A squeeze of lemon on your spinach salad, perhaps.

SNACKS

Many of us try to minimise snacking, but there are some nourishing snacks from which we can really reap benefit. Almonds are a great source of natural protein that can ease hunger. Since they contain high levels of magnesium, there's an added nutritional benefit: magnesium is a great anti-stress mineral.

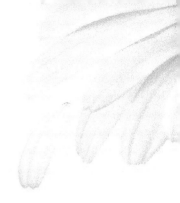

HAIR CARE PRODUCTS

INGREDIENTS TO AVOID

Hair washing would have to be the most confusing topic for women with hair loss. Apart from hair loss itself, that is.

Confusion is only fuelled further by the amount of conflicting advice we're given on how often to wash our hair and what to wash it with, especially when hair loss is a factor.

I used to wash my hair every other day, but it always looked best on wash day. Naturally, I planned my hair washing schedule around days when I wanted to look my best and days when it didn't matter as much. At that time, I used supermarket shampoos, choosing them based on nice packaging, delicious fragrances or discounted prices.

But once my hair started to fall out I realised I needed to choose quality. For a long while I mistakenly associated quality with price. I was paying exorbitant prices for hair salon shampoos and it took me a long time to work out that they made no difference at all. This was a point of major frustration for me – hair salon shampoo that cost the earth yet didn't seem to offer any benefit for my hair. Not only that, but some also seemed to make my hair drier and frizzier.

So-called volume and thickening shampoos make hair drier by design – frizzier hair **is** more voluminous. But the damage they can do is astounding. If our hair is thinning 'volume' is an attractive word for us. But we need to understand what that means in terms of the effects these products can have on our hair.

Over the years I have read countless scientific studies on female hair loss, shampoos, regrowth products, ingredients, long- and short-term damage. And yes, there are several ingredients that we must avoid when we're managing hair loss.

Parabens and sulfates

It's well known that we need to avoid these chemicals when choosing our hair products. But why?

Because parabens (used for cleansing and foaming in product formulations) can be absorbed through the skin and the scalp and studies have shown that they can disrupt normal hormonal cycles[54].

Sulfates are used as surfactants (sudsing agents) and are added to shampoos to remove dirt and dead skin cells from the scalp. But they can also be responsible for stripping the hair of its natural oils, making it dry and brittle. Dryness, itching, irritation and even hair loss often result from using products containing these nasties. Shampoos that contain sulfates are not recommended for dyed or bleached hair and should not be used on compromised hair also.

No wonder washing our hair every day with ordinary super-market shampoos can do such damage.

DMDM hydantoin

DMDM hydantoin has received a lot of publicity as a causative agent for hair loss. It is known as a formaldehyde releaser. That means, as it breaks down, over time, it gradually releases formaldehyde.[55]

DMDM hydantoin is used in many hair care products as a preservative.

Generally the amount of formaldehyde released is very small. However, many women swear it has caused hair loss for them, and it is known that this can cause allergic reactions such as a sore scalp, redness, itchiness and swelling in some individuals.[56]

The U.S. Food and Drug Administration website lists

DMDM hydantoin (1,3-dimethylol-5,5-dimethylhydantoin) as a common allergen found in cosmetic products.[57]

It is interesting to note that many of the large cosmetic companies and shampoo manufacturers have removed it from their formulations and make it very clear on their products and in their marketing that they do not contain DMDM hydantoin.

To be on the safe side check your shampoos, styling products and hair fibres and anything else you put on your hair to ensure this ingredient is not included.

MEA and DEA

Cocomide MEA and Cocomide DEA are added to cosmetics and shampoos as a surfactant and foam booster.

DEA may react with other ingredients in certain formulations to form a type of carcinogen. And both MEA and DEA have been linked with liver tumours.[58]

It is worth reading the ingredients list of the products you are using to ensure these ingredients are not included.

Petrochemicals

Petrochemicals are chemicals derived from petroleum (crude oil) or natural gas. There are petroleum and petroleum by-products in just about everything we put on our bodies, from creams to lotions, perfumes, lipsticks, nail polishes, eye shadows and of course, shampoos and conditioners.

According to the Campaign for Safe Cosmetics, when petroleum is properly refined it has no known health concerns.[59] However, when it has not been correctly refined it can be potentially harmful. The main health concern being cancer.

The only way you can be sure the petroleum ingredient in your shampoo is okay to use is if you can be sure it was refined properly. This requires the provision of a complete refining history.

Some jurisdictions insist on the refining history being provided prior to the use of these chemicals in cosmetic products. However others, like the USA do not.

When the petroleum is listed as 'fully refined as white petroleum' it is okay to use.

It would appear best to avoid products with petroleum or petroleum by-products in them unless the refined status is clearly shown.

So, what should we look for in a shampoo?

Firstly, look at the ingredient list on the label and avoid all of the ingredients above.

Then look at the same label for nourishing, natural ingredients that will nurture your hair such as:

- almond oil
- lavender oil
- peppermint oil

- orange oil
- rose oil
- jasmine oil
- green tea
- coffee bean extract
- coconut-based cleansers.

I spent a lot of time and effort sourcing shampoo and conditioner ingredients that are kind to hair, safe to use every day, and especially safe and nourishing to use on compromised hair.

The entire resulting Boost & Be range is free from nasties, packed with nourishing ingredients, made in Australia and kind to your hair.

The shampoo paradox

Have you ever noticed that a shampoo you initially love seems to stop working over time? This is a very common experience and there's a good reason for it.

When you first used and loved your new shampoo, it was most likely performing a specific purpose. For example, your hair may have been dry and brittle so you began using a moisturising shampoo and the effect was amazing. After using it for a while your hair is no longer as dry (thanks to the moisturising shampoo and conditioner) and so now, when you use a moisturising shampoo, it makes your hair feel greasy.

Other factors – such as a recent hair colour, a haircut (removing dry ends) or a lightening treatment growing out an inch or so – can also change the way your hair responds to various ingredients.

Shampoos and conditioners specifically designed to provide volume or thickness can make hair dry and brittle, especially if they are the type of volumising product that relies on drying the hair out to give the illusion of more volume. You may have initially loved the volume but now have hair that needs moisturising.

Some shampoos build up over time. Clarifying shampoos are great for clearing any build-up.

Whether you use one of the safe and kind-to-hair products I recommend or choose another brand for healthy hair growth, switching between formulations regularly will optimise your results.

pH and why it matters

You have probably heard about pH balanced shampoos and conditioners, and for good reason.

In order to understand the function of shampoo and its effect on the pH of hair you may need a quick reminder of some basic science.

pH is a scale that ranges from 1 to 14. A pH between 1 and 6 is acidic, 7 is considered neutral and a pH of 8 to 14 is alkaline.

To understand the effect of shampoo and conditioner on the hair. We need to focus on the pH balance of the hair shaft itself – the part of the hair that has left the skin surface and is no longer alive.

Given that we want to look after our hair so that its condition remains healthy for many years, we do need to take care of it by washing it with suitable products.

The hair shaft is made up of three main layers:

- the medulla (the inner layer)
- the cortex (the middle layer that surrounds the medulla)
- the cuticle (the outer, protective layer).

The cuticle helps the hair shaft to repel water and is instrumental in the cleaning and maintenance of healthy hair.

Normal, untreated hair has a pH of around 3.7 and the scalp has a normal pH of around 5.5.

According to a recent article in the *International Journal of Trichology*,[60] the majority of commercially available and supermarket shampoos have a pH of greater than 5, with some as high as 7 or 8.

Ultimately, these shampoos alter the natural pH of the hair, at which point the cuticle will open up and the hair shaft will become brittle. If the hair is then dried, it will have increased friction, causing frizz, hair breakage and hair tangling.

The main purpose of shampoo is to remove impurities from

the hair and the scalp. These impurities can not only adhere to the hair shaft (causing it to become heavy and limp) but also adhere to the scalp, where they can cause dermatitis, sebor-rhoea, alopecia or psoriasis.

To minimise friction and frizz it's important that a shampoo contains the right kind of cleansing agents, since the shampoo not only works on the scalp but also on the hair shaft. Surfactants are the cleaning agents in shampoo that have this effect.

As a side note, children's shampoos are usually neutral with a pH of around 7.0. This is a formulation strategy that enables a product to promote a 'no tears' claim. Although they may not cause eye irritation, these shampoos are not designed to condition the hair or the scalp and must definitely be avoided if you have dyed or bleached hair, or if your hair growth is compromised.

It's also important to understand the purpose of conditioner.

Since most shampoos alter the natural acidic state of the hair, they must be followed by a conditioner to return the pH to a healthy range. Conditioners are designed to neutralise electrostatic forces, eliminate the frizz effect, and close the cuticle by renormalising pH.

Avoiding conditioner leaves the hair at risk of breakage and likely to become tangled, knotted and static when dry, unless you are specifically using a shampoo with a pH lower than 5.5.

I talk to women all the time who are concerned that (since their hair seems to mostly shed during and after using condi-tioner) the conditioner is causing the shed.

Let me assure you that is definitely not the case. Rather, unless you brush your hair several times daily, hair in the shedding phase clings to the scalp and to other hairs until it gets the chance to fall away. Naturally this is more likely to happen when the hair is soft, smooth and slippery, as it is when slathered in conditioner.

Electrostatic charge

Another important aspect of shampoo and conditioner choices for women with hair loss is the electrostatic charge.

For women who use hair fibres the amount of cling derived from the product is crucial to the overall effect and success of the camouflage. Hair is naturally negatively charged. Cotton hair fibres like Boost N Blend are positively charged. Opposites attract and so the marriage of positive and negative charges is what creates the product hold and efficacy. By contrast, many keratin hair fibres are negatively charged, which is why they do not usually cling as well as cotton fibres.

Many factors can interrupt the negative charge of hair. For example using a shampoo without a conditioner, which can positively charge the hair. In that condition, hair fibres will not cling as well, if at all. Keep in mind that anti-dandruff shampoos tend to have a higher pH. We know that most of the commercial anti-dandruff shampoos, and some other treatment shampoos, affect the charge of the hair shaft. Again, if the hair shaft is not the correct pH, it will be prevented from attracting hair fibre products. In these circumstances many women complain that the hair fibre product they are using clumps on their scalp. The fibres they're using are not to blame though. It's their shampoo and conditioner, how often they use them and how effective their hair care techniques are.

Choosing your products

Could your shampoo be contributing to your hair loss?

Closely scrutinising the chemical additives we put **into** our bodies is an important health strategy but many of us forget to pay attention to the chemicals we put **on** our bodies.

A few years back mineral make-up swept the market by storm, offering a viable alternative to the chemical gunk that we'd been slathering on our faces for decades. More recently the health spotlight has turned to the hair care market.

What are natural hair care products like Boost & Be and are they worth the switch?

To quote one of the lovely ladies who wrote to me after trying our #KindToHair range:

> *My hair has completely changed since I started using the Boost & Be shampoos and conditioners. It's so much healthier and stronger. And I notice a lot less hair fall in the shower when I wash it. It actually has some shape now and I feel much less self-conscious about any visible scalp or my hair looking a bit dirty when it was*

freshly washed (anyone with flat, limp hair knows how that feels like).

Yep. We sure do!

But remember ladies, less hair fall in the shower is not due to some magical ingredient in this product (or any other shampoo or conditioner). It is most likely due to the passing of time which may have naturally resolved the issue. What can be attributed to this product though, is healthier and stronger hair.

NATURAL AND ORGANIC

Unlike most of the supermarket-aisle offerings, natural, organic and low-chemical shampoos and conditioners use essential oils, and plant and herb extracts to naturally cleanse and nourish the hair without exposing it to damaging chemicals.

Some of the positive and the negative aspects of natural, organic and low-chemical products are listed below.

Positive

- Safe for every day, and every other day, use
- No harmful chemicals
- Won't strip the hair of natural oils
- Won't interact with or strip synthetic hair colours
- Won't dry hair out and make it brittle and susceptible to breakage

- Safe for use on all hair types
- Safe for use by the whole family, children and pregnant or breastfeeding mothers included
- Usually smell amazing!

Negative

- Can be difficult to lather effectively without the chemical sodium lauryl sulfate which is contained in most common shampoos
- Often significantly more expensive than regular brands

Not labelled as natural or organic

Here I am referring to the (often rather cheap) supermarket and pharmacy brands. They usually contain synthetic chemical cleaning agents, some of which can cause problems for sensitive people. They also commonly contain the foaming chemical sodium lauryl sulfate, which is both irritating and damaging to the follicle.[61]

Some pros and cons of these products are listed below.

Positive

- Easy to lather
- Effective cleaning power
- Can be very cheap

Negative

- Contain sodium lauryl sulfate
- Often harmful to hair with regular use
- Strips hair of natural moisture, which can cause breakage (there is such a thing as 'too clean')
- Chemicals can irritate the scalp contributing to or exacerbating issues like dermatitis, dandruff and dry scalp.

It is well worth your time to search for natural and kind-to-hair products that are right for you. Read the ingredients lists – they will astound you.

INGREDIENTS THAT CAN HELP

There is a plethora of so-called hair growth shampoos on the market, containing a wide variety of mostly natural ingredients that are touted to assist in new hair growth.

When I was working on the Boost & Be shampoo range I spent a great deal of time researching ingredients that could optimise hair follicle health and thus support healthy hair growth.

Below are some of the popular healthy hair growth ingredients found in shampoos and other products, and what I discovered about their various claimed benefits.

Peppermint oil

According to a 2014 study, peppermint oil showed significant anti-inflammatory, antimicrobial and antifungal actions, as well as potent antioxidant activity and antiallergenic and anti-tumour effects.[62] That's a big wrap. And they're all actions we're looking for to improve compromised scalp health.

In the study conducted on mice, a very well-known hair growth stimulant called minoxidil (see later chapter on treatments) was compared to peppermint oil in a topical application. Both the peppermint oil and the minoxidil were applied at a 3% dilution to a shaved area once a day, six days a week for four weeks. From week 2, peppermint oil grew hair more rapidly compared to minoxidil. After four weeks the peppermint oil showed a considerably rapid increase in hair growth when compared to the minoxidil.

And that's not all – increases in skin thickness, follicle depth, number, and measurable hair growth were observed at each investigation point, suggesting that peppermint oil is more effective than minoxidil as a topical application for hair growth.

Personally, I experienced a significant increase in hair growth when using peppermint oil as a topical ingredient. That's why it became one of the key ingredients in a Boost & Be shampoo.

Not only is peppermint oil an effective hair-health ingredient – it feels refreshing and stimulating to the scalp and smells divine. Like all natural ingredients it's the consistent use over time that creates great results.

Rosemary oil

I have not found any conclusive studies on rosemary oil and its effect on hair growth, specifically for women. It does have a strong traditional reputation as a scalp stimulant and may certainly help, without the side effects of conventional treatments like minoxidil.

According to Medical News Today, a 2013 study conducted on mice found that rosemary oil could regrow their hair.[63] It was reported that 'although this study was not conclusive, the authors theorise that rosemary oil might prevent dihydrotestosterone (DHT) from binding to hormone receptors that enable it to attack the hair follicles'.

I would consider rosemary oil a relevant therapeutic ingredient for a specific type of hair loss that's caused by an excess of DHT on the scalp. You may recall that DHT is an androgen hormone converted from testosterone, found in skin and hair follicles in much larger quantities in men than in women. When it is found on the scalp in excess amounts it is associated with a thinning of hair follicles, which influences hair growth.

Many shampoos formulated for male hair loss contain known DHT blockers. But before you reach for one consider that unless your hair loss is caused by an overabundance of DHT on your scalp, it will likely not be effective.

Caffeine

In theory caffeine has the capacity to counteract DHT's negative effects by reducing the production of certain harmful proteins, improving blood flow and reducing inflammation. All these actions are critical for improving hair health.

There's a lot of debate in the medical world as to whether caffeine shampoos have the capacity to replicate the results of laboratory testing. At this stage caffeine shampoos are generally not endorsed as an effective hair-growth solution, mainly due to a lack of solid evidence. Because of the DHT-blocking action, shampoos containing caffeine are marketed to men.

While the topical application of caffeine may help improve hair growth where there is a DHT causation, unfortunately your morning latte will not have the same effect.

A 2007 German study showed some evidence that caffeine stimulates follicles and activates hair growth under laboratory conditions, its main function working to block DHT.[64]

Saw palmetto

Saw palmetto is a traditional herbal tonic for men, known for its anti-inflammatory effects, for improving urinary tract health and as a testosterone booster.

There is limited research on the effectiveness of saw palmetto in preventing hair loss, even though this is one of the herb's main indications in traditional herbal medicine. It certainly does seem to slow down hair loss in men when they take it orally at a good dose over time, again by blocking the production of DHT. Saw palmetto is also a common ingredient in shampoos marketed to promote male hair growth, as a limited study did point to some hair growth benefits on topical application.[65]

Women who suffer from androgen-induced hair loss may benefit from taking saw palmetto orally or using it topically but there is no solid research to confirm its use.

Saw palmetto is also a common ingredient in hair-growth shampoos marketed to women. If inflammation and excess DHT are involved in your hair loss, you certainly may see improved growth over time with this ingredient.

Nettle (aka stinging nettle root, *Urtica dioica*)

This plant has been widely and traditionally used as a treatment for benign prostatic hyperplasia due to its ability to inhibit the conversion of testosterone to DHT. However at this point clinical trials on its efficacy in hair loss are sadly lacking. Nettle has been studied in combination with other herbal extracts, where the combination was shown to support new hair growth.[66]

If nettle is an ingredient in the shampoo you are using, then you may find it beneficial as an addition to a solid therapeutic formulation.

Provitamin B5

Provitamin B5 (panthenol) is one of the most popular ingredients in hair care products around the world. Used in shampoo formulations as a weightless volumiser, it doesn't dry out the hair in the way that many other volumising ingredients do.

One of the few vitamins that is able to penetrate into the lower skin layers, vitamin B5 can be absorbed by the skin cells. It is known as a deeply moisturising ingredient, depositing its nourishing effects deep into the cortex of the hair.

Look for shampoos containing panthenol; it's a boon for hair health and volume.

Keratin

There's been a lot of buzz about keratin in the hair-growth industry in recent years. It's been touted as a miracle ingredient, able to smooth curls and frizz while adding body and shine.

But is it really all it's cracked up to be? Is keratin good or bad for thinning hair? The marketing would have us believe that the keratin used in hair products (like keratin hair fibres, keratin smoothing treatments and keratin shampoos and conditioners) is the same keratin that makes up our hair and nails.

This is only partially true.

Keratin is a family of fibrous structural proteins, and humans have 54 functioning keratin genes. Only some of these keratin genes are found in human hair and they are not likely to exactly mimic the keratins found in hair products.

Where does keratin come from?

As well as being present in human hair, keratin is also found in the wool, horns, feathers, claws and hooves of animals. It is from these sources that many keratin hair product manufacturers obtain their keratin. So, while you may believe that you are buying something that closely resembles or even imitates human hair, you are likely to be buying a product that contains an animal source of keratin.

Does this really matter?

Extracting keratin from animal parts makes keratin an animal protein, which means it naturally contains a large amount of bacteria. In order to render it safe and hygienic by strict cosmetic standards, significant amounts of bactericides and preservatives are added to the formula.

Enter . . . more chemicals.

Are all keratin hair products made from animal protein?

Not all, but most are.

Unfortunately, the products that are not made from animal protein aren't any healthier. The alternative way to produce keratin is to synthesise it by mixing chemicals that imitate the structure of the forms of keratin found in human hair. These types of keratin products are chemical cocktails, not natural products.

Are keratin hair products harmful?

No, not usually.

However, if you notice any concerning changes in your health while using keratin hair products, perhaps it would be a good idea to cease using the product. If you read hair-loss forums, you may have seen some people reporting side effects such as breathing difficulties and skin and eye irritations resulting from using keratin products.

The main chemicals to be wary of in keratin hair products are ammonium chloride, DMDM hydantoin and formaldehyde. These are commonly used in keratin hair products and known to be harmful for some people, even in small quantities.[67]

Is there a way to 'boost' natural keratin stores?

As keratin is a protein you may find that increasing the protein in your diet could assist in preventing or slowing hair loss. Studies have shown that many women are not eating enough protein from healthy daily sources. Since your body needs protein to make hair strong, a lack of it may be contributing to fine, thin or thinning hair.

What about keratin hair fibres?

Keratin hair fibres are usually derived from animal proteins. One of the major brands boasts that their keratin comes from wool and another clearly states they use DMDM hydantoin in their formulation. Another well-known brand has a long list of chemicals on their label.

Are there any alternatives to keratin fibres?

Cotton fibres are plant based. They don't require a huge number of chemical additives and are safe even for the most sensitive people. Online reviews suggest that the cotton products have superior aesthetic results as well as health and environmental benefits, so you may find you prefer them.

Hair fibre solutions like Boost N Blend are made from natural cotton, with not one keratin hair fibre or animal source in sight.

DRY SHAMPOO

Dry shampoo can feel like a real game changer.

On days when we don't have time to wash, dry or style our hair, or we need a quick fix between sweaty gym workouts, reaching for a dry shampoo offers a solution for soaking up oil and cleaning our hair, water-free. But few people know that dry shampoo has the potential to damage hair health and contribute to thinning hair and hair loss.

Take a moment to look at the ingredients. No doubt you will see a long list of chemicals that you do not want to put anywhere near your compromised hair, scalp and follicles.

It is a common misconception that washing your hair every day results in increased hair loss, leading many women to reach for dry shampoos as a 'safe' alternative. The truth is that avoiding daily hair washing, particularly by using a dry shampoo, does far more damage than frequent cleansing with a quality wet shampoo and good technique. If your hair is thinning you are far better off washing your hair every day and keeping it looking fresh and bouncy naturally than using a dry shampoo.

Bad news for dry shampoo users

From dermatologists to trichologists to hairdressers, industry experts agree that excessive use of dry shampoo can lead to a host of hair and scalp problems including:[68] [69]

- **Dull hair colour with a lack of shine:** Most dry shampoos contain powdered ingredients like aluminium starch and corn starch which appear matte when applied to the hair. Those who colour their hair tend to be fearful of stripping out the colour with wet shampoos but dry shampoos have the same effect. Ultimately the colour in your hair looks less shiny and healthy if you overuse dry shampoo products.
- **An increase in dryness and dandruff:** Dry shampoos are designed to draw moisture and oil away from the scalp. It follows that excess use will cause a dry and flaky scalp. This is especially harmful if you already suffer from dryness and your hair and scalp tend to react to products.

- **A build-up of dead skin, germs and bacteria:** The scalp is simply an extension of the skin on your face. We know from experience that an oily, dirty build-up on facial skin leads to clogged pores, blemishes and breakouts. The same is true of the skin on your scalp. Imagine powdering your face for a few days without washing it . . . Don't do this to your scalp.
- **Blocked hair follicles and disrupted hair cycles:** Blocked follicles go hand in hand with a build-up of dirt and bacteria. This clogging effect may disrupt the natural, healthy hair cycle.
- **Scalp cysts and acne:** Blocked follicles are vulnerable to infection. When bacteria is trapped in the follicles, cysts and scalp pimples can develop.
- **Tangled tresses:** The drying effect of dry shampoos can lead to tangled and fragile hair shafts. Combing through these knots can result in breakage or lead to healthy hairs being pulled out unnecessarily.

Tips for thinning hair

- Switch to a detergent-free shampoo that will clean the hair thoroughly without disrupting the protective barrier. These products ideally remove excess dirt and styling products but not healthy, natural oils. Look for a range that is gentle, nourishing and deep cleansing, especially for women with thinning hair.

- Use a natural hair-loss concealer made from cotton fibres that will gently absorb excess oil without drying your hair and will have a similar effect to dry shampoo in boosting root volume. The Boost N Blend range of hair fibres for women is available in a variety of natural shades.
- Use charcoal hair-drying tissues (portable, oil-absorbing sheets, infused with tapioca starch and activated black charcoal powder) to absorb excess oil.

And, my most important piece of advice . . .

WASH YOUR HAIR EVERY DAY

If your hair is not shedding you may find that your regrowth rate is slow to non-existent.

Washing your hair every day will stimulate your hair follicles and promote healthy growth. I have seen it many times, both in my own experience and in the thousands of women I help through my work. New hair growth slowed to a virtual halt at a certain point in my hair loss journey. Although I wasn't shedding any longer, I wasn't growing any new hair either. I started to wash my hair every day with a detergent-free shampoo that contained peppermint oil and within three months I had significant new hair growth all over my scalp.

My tip for all women struggling with hair loss is to choose a high quality shampoo that does not contain any nasty detergents and is bursting with healthy ingredients, like the #KindToHair Boost & Be range. And to use it daily.

WHAT IF MY HAIR IS DRY AND BREAKING?

If all this talk of dry hair is hitting home there are some additional hair care strategies that may help you:

1. Between shampooing and conditioning: towel dry your hair. Just as face cream applied to a wet face won't be well absorbed – the same goes for your hair.
2. Use a hair dryer to partially dry your hair before applying your styling products as this will help the product gain better absorption.
3. Resist the temptation to rub your hair vigorously when towel drying. You can do a lot of damage to wet hair as it is more likely to stretch and break. Blot and dab as your technique. Try a specially designed microfibre hair- towel wrap

for women with thinning hair. There is one in the Boost N Blend range.

4. Never use a brush or fine-tooth comb on wet hair. Wet hair is slightly elastic and can break very easily. Always use a broad-tooth comb and be especially gentle with wet hair.

How to wash your hair

The aim for 'squeaky clean' was a hard habit for me to break!

When I was a teenager and learning to wash my hair, articles in all the magazines I read told me I should wash my hair until it was squeaky clean. This was fine advice for my young, thick, healthy hair. But once I found myself facing hair loss, I realised I needed to drop the habit. Hair doesn't need to be squeaky to be clean; in fact, this usually indicates over washing or a harsh product. Your hair simply needs to be washed regularly and with good technique.

Shampooing

When you select shampoos that are kind to your hair (without all the nasty foaming and sudsing ingredients) you may also find that it is harder to get a good lather. The reason for this is simple: harsh detergents (surfactants) lather up very easily. Milder and gentler surfactants do not.

A great habit to establish is washing your hair thoroughly with water first – before you apply shampoo. This helps in two ways. Firstly, it helps rinse away any product, dust and grime as an initial step. Secondly, it helps to saturate the hair shafts so that your shampoo can coat and cleanse all the strands. This step also helps to create a better lather in a gentle shampoo.

When you rinse your hair don't aim for the 'squeak'. Get to know how it feels when your hair has been cleansed effectively, but not over-cleansed. Most shampoo manufacturers recommend you shampoo twice. I echo this advice, although I don't always do a second wash. If I wash my hair every day, or it's getting too dry, I skip the second cleanse. You will get to know what's right for you, too.

Conditioning

You now know that applying conditioner is a vital part of effective and healthy hair washing in order to balance pH. Understanding how to apply it for optimal results is another matter.

In order to give conditioner the best possible chance to work on your hair, it is better if your hair is not dripping wet when you apply it.

Just as we dry our faces before applying moisturiser to optimise absorption, I recommend towel drying between the shampooing and conditioning steps. If this sounds like too much effort, hear me out!

Hair towels, like the Boost N Blend microfibre towels, are light and easy to hang. You can place one on the outside of the shower handle or door handle, or sling it over the bath or the top of the shower wall so it can be easily reached. A soft hand towel will also do. After shampooing, poke your head out from the water stream and give it a quick pat dry – it only takes a few seconds to take off the bulk of the water.

You will find that your conditioner clings better to the hair for longer, giving it the chance to absorb well and do its job properly.

Comb conditioner through if you like and always leave it in for a few minutes before rinsing if you have time to spare. If you have a scalp massager, use it at this point. One way to stimulate your follicles is to massage them. Every day if you can.

When it's time to rinse out your conditioner, aim to cleanse it gently away until you can no longer feel the slippery texture of it in your hair rather than achieve the 'squeak'.

Aim for soft and silky, not squeaky.

Nourishing hair masks

Introduce a nourishing mask as part of your regimen. The Boost & Be Repair Mask is low in chemicals, kind to hair and offers exceptional hydration to damaged and dry hair.

There are many hair masks on the market today for good reason – they can do wonders for your hair. Some are required to leave in overnight, which I just can't imagine doing, or being good for thinning hair. Much better to find one that offers its benefits in 10 minutes and apply it just before washing. You can also use a mask in place of conditioner every now and then to keep your hair nourished and moisturised.

The Boost & Be Repair Mask is great for this purpose. Just ten minutes before washing is nourishing and helps to keep the frizz at bay.

HAIRSTYLES FOR THINNING HAIR

GOING PLATINUM?

Platinum hair trends come and go but it's not just for the rich and famous.

While many celebrities are embracing platinum just to stay on trend, some are simply savvy women who have cottoned on to the advantages of platinum hair and they couldn't be happier.

Going platinum if you're going grey

It can be time consuming, expensive and downright annoying to constantly dye away your grey roots. But if you have darker hair they're too visible to ignore. It is well worth considering the relative freedom of platinum-coloured hair. Greys will blend seamlessly into this spectacular colour and you can neglect the salon for long periods of time while still looking your best. In fact, many salon colourists recommend platinum hair as a transitional strategy for women embracing their silver.

Going platinum if your hair is thinning

If you suffer from hair loss and have light-coloured skin, you're probably more than aware that your scalp is visible through your hair. You may have tried endless styling products and hairstyles to hide that pink or lily-white scalp. Here's where the camouflaging of platinum hair could work for you.

Platinum hair is much closer to most pale skin colours than darker shades, so the contrast between your scalp and platinum blonde hair will appear much less obvious. Pair this with a platinum hair fibre concealer and you'll have thicker, on-trend hair with no visible scalp to concern you.

If you have darker skin then the platinum look can and does look absolutely stunning. While there is more contrast between the hair and skin, the use of platinum hair fibres will provide the perfect coverage in moments. A few shakes and visible scalp skin disappears.

While considering this option, keep in mind that going lighter always involves stripping colour from the hair which can lead to dry, brittle hair. Best if you are going to do this, to consciously use a good quality shampoo and conditioner and a nourishing mask if needed.

STYLE CHOICES

Avoid a straight part

Parting the hair in a straight line, whether at the centre or the side, makes the hair gap appear wider on women with thinning hair and is not a recommended styling option.

Have you ever admired the zigzag part used by many famous models and actresses in magazine shoots? These creative part lines are not just for celebrities – you can easily style them yourself.

Play around with your part. If you are using hair fibres, apply a little to your usual part line. Then, using a comb, make your zigzag before applying a little more of the fibres. Use your fingers to pat or 'fluff' it in and admire your result.

Short hair

Women often send me photos of their thinning hair and one thing I commonly notice is that their chosen style is simply too long. If your hair is thinning your goal is to create the impression of more volume. It might seem as if longer hair equates to thicker hair but usually the opposite visual effect is achieved. When thinning hair is long it drags hair downwards so that it sits closer to the top of the head, exposing the scalp. Further, the visual effect of long, thin hair gives a more obvious impression of a lack of volume.

It may challenge your comfort zone but, seriously, consider trying a shorter style. Once your hair is shorter (and lighter), it will be easier to lift away from your scalp – that's what creates visual volume. Then apply Boost N Blend hair fibre concealer to your hair, near your scalp. With less weight and drag, your hair will appear significantly thicker.

A blunt cut

Blunt hair cuts really do give the aesthetic impression of thicker hair.

When all your hair ends sharply in one straight line, a fuller effect is achieved. When thin hair is layered, it can look even thinner at the ends.

Discuss your options for blunt cuts with a trusted stylist the next time you feel like a change.

Avoid back-combing

Back-combing or teasing your hair at the roots does have the effect of lifting your hair, and with the use of a cotton hair fibre concealer it will appear thicker.

But be careful with this technique. If your hair tends to fall out, heavy back-combing over a long period of time can worsen the problem.

After applying your hair fibre concealer, use one hand to lift your hair at the roots and spray under the hair with a quality firm-hold hairspray. This trick can help to keep your hair looking bouncy and 'camera-ready' all day long.

TIPS FOR SUMMER

Whether it's from sun, sand or surf, our hair can take quite a beating over the summer months.

Here are some quick tips to help you survive the hot season with thinning hair.

Sunscreen

Many of us have a widening part or visible scalp and while we may be painfully aware of the aesthetic drawbacks of the issue, we may not have thought about the potential health consequences.

One of the key biological roles our hair plays is protecting our scalp from the sun, so those areas not fully covered by hair are at risk of sun damage. It's a good idea to wear a hat whenever possible or tie your hair up to cover the gaps. But these two looks may not be what you had in mind for the summer BBQ.

So, a quick tip: apply sunscreen to a cotton bud and carefully apply it to areas of visible scalp. This will protect your scalp against harsh UV rays without making your hair greasy. You can also make sure you have good coverage with a hair fibre concealer. Along with a zigzag part line, which also provides some protection, you'll create some fabulous, fresh looks.

Rinse hair in fresh water after chlorine or saltwater swimming

Cooling off in the pool or at the beach is one of the best things about summer but our hair may not agree.

Both salt and chlorinated water can dry hair out and lead to damage and breakage. Of course, it's possible to swim without getting your hair wet but that's not the most fun or practical option.

To mitigate water damage simply rinse your hair with fresh water as soon as you can and then shampoo and condition with nourishing products later.

Hair care for summer

With the extra sun exposure, the pool and the surf, our hair has the potential to become extra dry during the summer months. To protect against brittleness and dryness stock up on high quality treatments and leave-in conditioners to minimise breakage. Some hair care companies also make UV protection sprays, which can specifically protect from sun damage.

Sun visors

If you want to wear a hat to protect your face, but want to avoid 'hat hair', a sun visor can be an excellent option.

This also has the aesthetic bonus of covering any thinning areas towards the front of your head. Just remember to use the cotton bud sunscreen method if you go with this look.

HELPER HAIR

A hair topper, also known as a crown extension, is a hair piece that clips into the existing hair to make hair look fuller and/ or longer, or to cover thinning areas. Hair toppers come with built-in clips that slide into existing hair on the top of the head and simply snap into place. A hair topper is almost always bought in the same colour and style as the existing hair so that the addition of the topper is visually seamless. A hair salon can colour and style a hair topper to fit even more perfectly with your current style and colour.

Some toppers offer a fringe or bangs too, offering a risk-free style option. Both human-hair toppers and synthetic options can be straightened and curled just like natural hair. Hair toppers come in a variety of colours and lengths and can be shampooed for cleanliness and maintenance.

For women with hair loss a topper is an easy fix for thinning hair or visible scalp areas. Toppers can also provide a fun and instant hair transformation and are great fun for special occasions like weddings and parties. Many celebrities wear toppers on screen and in photo shoots – they're not just for women with hair loss.

A wig is a full head of hair usually woven onto a cap made of cotton or nylon. The hairs are woven together into wefts, which are then sewn onto the cap. The cap is worn over the whole head, entirely covering the hair underneath.

Wigs can be very useful while women are undergoing (or have recently gone through) chemotherapy, or when hair loss has reached a certain point without successful treatment. You will know when that is.

Wigs can be made from human hair or synthetic hair fibres. When wearing a wig the natural hair sits under the wig cap when it is placed on the head. Wigs come in a variety of styles and colours and are generally quite easy to fit. Wigs are generally more expensive than hair toppers. They're not always a practical option for swimming, exercising or spending time at the beach and some women complain that wigs can become hot and itchy.

Whether you're searching for human-hair wigs, synthetic wigs or the best clip-on hair topper you can find, there's quite a bit to consider before you decide.

Will a topper or a wig suit me best?

Women choose their hair piece depending on many different factors: cost, length, the coverage they require, and where they are in their hair loss journey. Women with hair loss associated with alopecia areata or chemotherapy often prefer a full coverage wig, while women with naturally fine or thinning hair, or those experiencing FPHL or shedding, more often choose to wear synthetic or human-hair toppers to help create a fuller look. Both options are great for women wanting to enhance their hair and looking for more coverage.

Cost

The price of a wig varies depending on the type of hair (human or synthetic), number of wefts, style, colour and length. Synthetic pieces are generally cheaper due to the higher availability and lower cost of synthetic fibres.

How long do hair helpers last?

Human-hair toppers can last anywhere from 4 to 12 months with daily wear.

Human-hair wigs, depending on how well they are maintained, can last up to three years, while synthetic wigs last up to a year. The better you look after your wig, the longer it will last. There are several tutorials online to help you style and maintain them with good technique.

PREVENTING HAIR LOSS

While it may sound too good to be true, if you're a woman who has female hair loss in your family, there are some strategies that will minimise the likelihood of the same problem coming your way. Likewise, if you are suffering from hair loss and you have daughters, then this will be great advice to pass on to them. And if you have had hair loss in the past, this advice will help to prevent future occurrences.

NUTRIENTS AND DIET

You know the saying: 'You only get out what you put in!'

Well, it applies to the health of your hair just as much as working hard in your career or hitting the gym.

In order to have healthy hair it's important to have a healthy body. There are countless vitamins, minerals and other nutrients that are essential for healthy hair, covered in earlier sections of this book. A diagnosed deficiency in any one of them can cause hair loss. Remember that it's important never to guess what you may be deficient in as taking supplemental nutrients you don't need can be harmful. Visit your doctor for advice.

As well as ensuring that you are getting enough vitamins and minerals, there are a few foods (see the sections on iron and protein) that you should make sure you include in your diet to help prevent the onset of hair loss and to nourish your body and overall health.

BLOOD TESTS AND GENERAL CHECK-UPS

It's impossible to know for sure if you're deficient in any nutrient if you don't get a blood test. Healthy individuals under 35 should get a full blood test every two to three years, while those over 35 or with any known illnesses or deficiencies should get a blood test annually.

Unfortunately, many doctors are resistant to ordering more than the basic blood test. Ideally you would get your full iron panel, thyroid, hormone, vitamins D and B as a minimum.

AVOID OVER-STYLING

Traction alopecia is a form of gradual hair loss that occurs when the hair is constantly pulled in tight braiding styles, tight ponytails (and man buns). It's important to avoid any style that pulls tightly on the roots of the hair if you are vulnerable to hair loss.

Additionally, overuse of heated styling appliances like flat irons and curlers can cause damage to the hair, causing it to break and fall. If you must 'fry' your hair, make sure you use a heat protection spray and try not to do it every day.

It's a good idea to keep styling products to a minimum and, as much as possible, use kind-to-hair products like those I have recommended. Be sure to gently wash them out and definitely don't try to brush them out.

CHOOSE HIGH QUALITY HAIR PRODUCTS

Natural and organic hair care products can be more expensive than their cheap chemical counterparts but if you're worried about hair loss they are an important investment. Mainstream chemical-laden shampoos and conditioners can cause irritation and dryness by stripping the hair of its natural oils. They can even cause harm with long-term use. If you can't make the switch to natural and organic hair care products, select salon-quality products from your hairdresser – anything you find in the supermarket aisle is simply 'junk food for hair.'

Natural really is best!

TREATMENTS

Treating hair loss in a woman is a complex process and one which many general physicians find puzzling, for good reason. Discovering the root cause when there are so many options, and then considering underlying health issues and the many possible triggers, makes the decision about how to treat the issue all the more baffling.

Is there a cure?

If there was a single 'cure' for female hair loss, I would have already written a book about it.

The harsh truth of the matter is that while there are plenty of scientists doing great work to find a cure for hair loss – and there is some hope – there are only a few trials that have shown promise so far.

In this section I list some of the potential solutions that many report **do** make a difference.

The first place to start is in diagnosing and correcting any underlying health issues such as nutritional deficiencies, and thyroid, gut and hormone issues. Then look at triggers, recent illness, weight fluctuations, medications both long- and short-term, supplements being taken, and then external sources such as physical damage done to the hair and scalp. Scalp issues too need to be diagnosed or ruled out.

While the underlying causes and triggers are being addressed, there are a number of ways that you can directly change the way hair loss progresses. These come in two different treatment types – stimulants and blockers – as well as more invasive surgical procedures.

Stimulants work on the hair follicle in a number of different ways, depending on the stimulant. They stimulate the follicle to encourage hair growth. Stimulants can be either topical (applied directly to the follicle) or taken orally as a medication.

Blockers work to block the androgen receptors on the scalp, which then prevents DHT from acting on the follicles to slow and eventually prevent hair growth through the process of miniaturisation. These tend to work better on men due to the fact that male pattern hair loss is generally caused by an excess of DHT. While an excess of DHT also can cause hair loss in women, it is less prevalent in women and therefore blockers are less likely to be effective on women.

Invasive procedures refer to any type of treatment that requires some kind of surgical intervention. Most of these procedures involve a local anaesthetic and possibly some form of light sedation, and a consultation with a hair transplant surgeon in a hair loss clinic.

STIMULANTS

Minoxidil (Rogaine, Regaine)

Minoxidil is a stimulant treatment. It is a safe hair loss medication that works by stimulating the hair follicle. It is scientifically proven to be effective for hair loss and is prescribed for both male and female hair loss the world over.

While the most common brand names for minoxidil are Regaine and Rogaine, it is also sold under other brand names and is included as an ingredient in many hair stimulant products including hair drops and oils.

Minoxidil is approved by the Australian Therapeutic Goods Administration and the US Food and Drug Administration, and no doubt similar organisations around the world, for use in the treatment of hair loss. It has proven to be completely safe with minimal side effects and it is available over the counter. If there were concerning side effects, minoxidil wouldn't be approved for self-administration.

Even though it's been on the market now for over 35 years, doctors and scientists still do not know exactly how minoxidil works. We do know that it is a vasodilator, meaning that it opens up the blood vessels, thus increasing blood flow and therefore the availability of oxygen and nutrients to the area to which it is topically applied.

Although minoxidil can be taken as a tablet, here I am referring to the application of minoxidil as a liquid or foam which is applied directly to the hair follicles. Note that when applied topically it is not applied to the hair, it must be applied in direct contact with the scalp.

Minoxidil is a long-term therapy, not a cure. It doesn't address the underlying cause of the hair loss, but it does boost growth, largely by improving the health and quality of the hair that the follicle produces. You need to use minoxidil for as long as you want to treat your issue – it is dose dependent, much like a blood pressure tablet. You don't just take a blood pressure tablet for a few months and expect the problem to go away, unless you are working on improving the underlying conditions causing the high blood pressure. You understand that the treatment needs to be maintained for as long as you need to achieve the result. Minoxidil is the same.

How does this treatment work? As we know, after a hair is shed a new one grows in its place some three months later. Minoxidil works on that new hair to increase its diameter so that, over time, the miniaturising of the hair shaft reduces, and the hair shaft can grow through physically thicker.

Since minoxidil also elongates the growth (anagen) phase, the shedding phase will also be decreased and for most women shedding will significantly slow.

Some women see an increase in shedding **initially** with minoxidil, which is to be expected. For a new hair to grow, the old hair needs to be shed, much like losing baby teeth. Consider the way a baby tooth gets wobbly only when there is a new one underneath it ready to push it out: hair is similar. If you experience a big shed after starting minoxidil it can be a good sign that it's working and that there are many new hairs underneath getting ready to grow through.

These new hairs will ideally be marginally thicker. But be mindful that visible thickening may take many months to result. For a start, it will be at least three months before any new hairs begin to grow where the old hairs were shed. One of the other expected results of minoxidil treatment is a slowing down of the progression of hair loss. You will notice that the miniaturisation and gradual loss of hair will stop where it was when you started the therapy and over time the hair shaft should start to thicken up, provided you continue the treatment. Stay the course. It will be worth it.

Miniaturisation

You can expect to begin to see some results from minoxidil treatment in four to six months at the earliest. Realistically, it may take closer to a year to see tangible results, which will be even more impressive at two years of treatment.

Be mindful that not everyone achieves great results with minoxidil. Approximately 40% of women will see obvious benefit by way of an increase in follicle diameter, occasionally a small increase in the number of hairs and definitely a decrease in shedding (after a possible initial shedding).

Another 40% will see a cessation of the deterioration of the follicle, so the gradual thinning will cease over time – no new hair, not much of an increase in density, but no more loss.[70] [71]

Remember also that the gradual thinning and aging of hair is progressive, so the sooner you begin treatment with minoxidil the sooner you can halt the progression.

Using minoxidil

Minoxidil comes in a liquid or a foam. The liquid tends to create more of a reaction in sensitive scalps because it contains propylene glycol as a preservative, which can cause itching, dry scalp and flaking. Another common complaint about the liquid is that it makes styling hair difficult as it can create a 'sticky' feeling. The liquid is absorbed by the skin in around 60 to 90 minutes so you do need to leave it on for at least that long. Given that time frame, you could reasonably put it on overnight and wash your hair in the morning. The foam option tends to be better tolerated than the liquid, and doesn't cause the sticky feeling. It only takes around 15 minutes to soak in so you can apply it just before you wash your hair.

While the label recommends that minoxidil is applied twice a day, the active ingredient is known to remain on the scalp for up to 21 hours. So once a day is usually enough.

According to Dr Russell Knudson, an Australian hair transplant surgeon, although the label suggests 1ml per application, you need to apply as much as is required to fully cover the area you are treating, which can vary widely from person to person.[72] The best advice would seem to be to apply as much as is needed to cover the area of the scalp where you hope to improve your hair, and to do so once a day.

There is also an oral minoxidil which requires a doctor's prescription. It does tend to have side effects, which are best discussed with your doctor or specialist.

Minoxidil, washing and styling

I get asked how to use minoxidil with styling and haircare products frequently. If you follow the advice here and apply it once a day at night, then it will be easily washed out in the morning. If you don't wash your hair daily it will be completely dry by the morning.

If you are a cotton hair fibre user then you need to be sure you are applying the fibres to completely dry hair and scalp. Don't worry about applying the minoxidil in an area where you have fibres. Depending on how much cotton fibre product you apply, you can simply brush the fibres aside with your fingers or a comb and apply the minoxidil in that area before you go to bed. Reapply the fibres onto your dry hair and scalp in the morning.

I almost invariably advocate more hair washing rather than less. If you are using minoxidil in addition to hair fibres then frequent washing would be preferable.

Low-level laser therapy

A number of clinical studies have been carried out on low-level laser therapy (LLLT) for both men and women with hair loss. Not surprisingly, more on men than on women.[73]

I was able to find a study carried out exclusively on healthy females between the ages of 18 to 60. All had been diagnosed with androgenic alopecia. The results appear very encouraging with 51% of the women showing an increase in hair count [74].

It is well established that infrared light promotes tissue repair and stimulates cell activity. It has also shown beneficial effects in the treatment of stroke, joint pain, nerve regeneration and wound healing. Since we know that hair loss happens at the cellular level in the hair follicle, it stands to reason that anything that can stimulate follicle cells will have a positive effect in treating some types of hair loss.

LLLT is approved by the FDA for the treatment of both male and female hair loss. This is a significant fact considering there are only two drugs approved by the FDA for the treatment of hair loss; minoxidil and finasteride[75]. Although noting that finasteride is only approved for the treatment of hair loss in men.

There are two main ways to receive laser therapy: at a hair loss clinic or at home using a laser device.

While attending a hair loss clinic is ideal, you would need to attend at least three times per week for many months to see any real benefit. This can be cost and time prohibitive for many people.

In recent years there has been a surge in at-home, light-weight and very portable devices that allow you to use laser treatment in the privacy of your own home, when it suits you and at a fraction of the price of clinic treatments.

Laser caps, bands, combs and helmets are all on offer, and at-home equipment is improving rapidly. Since it appears that frequency of application is a key factor in achieving the best results, at-home options appear to me to be the best choice in laser treatment.

However, *caveat emptor* – buyer beware. There appear to be a huge number of low- cost devices that most likely do not have the technology and power to deliver therapeutic levels of laser therapy. The cost associated with these devices appears to be in line with the quality of the delivery mechanism. You get what you pay for.

Clinical trials of LLLT seem to point to a certain number of laser diodes and a specific wattage being optimal for results. The number of laser diodes in the cap, the wattage of the delivery and the resulting depth of subcutaneous tissue penetration by the laser are all factors that produce differing results.[76]

There are some very high quality laser caps available that have a portable battery and can be worn outside the house – perhaps perfect to wear while on a morning walk? The ideal length of time for wear seems to vary depending on the device but something in the order of 30 to 45 minutes three or four times a week seems to be a common instruction.

Note that LLLT is a form of stimulating therapy, like minoxidil although it works via a completely different mechanism. Minoxidil works as a vasodilator while LLLT works on cell regeneration. So it would appear that using both together would deliver the best and quickest results and is generally regarded as very safe.

As with all hair loss treatments, for optimal results you will need to get to the bottom of your underlying causes and work on holistic healing and health while using treatment strategies.

BLOCKERS

Spironolactone and cyproterone acetate (CPA)

Both spironolactone and cyproterone acetate are anti-androgenic pharmaceutical drugs that many dermatologists are now prescribing for women with hair loss.

Spironolactone is often combined with minoxidil as a treatment for FPHL.

An interesting study was published in the *British Journal of Dermatology* in 2005 comparing two anti-androgenic therapies: spironolactone and cyproterone acetate.[77] When the study concluded there was no significant difference in the results between the two therapies so the results were combined. It was noted that 88% of the women who received either of these anti-androgens could expect to see no progression of their hair loss **nor any improvement**. In other words, the problem halted but did not reverse.

This was a limited study and the author suggested that further study was required including a study which included a placebo-controlled group.

Spironolactone has been used in the treatment of FPHL for over 20 years. During its broad use as a diuretic it was accidentally discovered that spironolactone improved hirsutism – a dominance of male hormones in a woman that causes, among other things, hair growth in a male pattern on the face and body. Spironolactone was found to reduce the production of androgens (male hormones) and was also seen to block androgen receptors. For this reason, spironolactone has been prescribed to women with hair loss. Some clinicians report a cessation of hair loss in women and others have seen partial hair growth in some women taking spironolactone.

A more recent study was conducted in 2014 on a small sample of women with acne and androgenic alopecia who were treated with cyproterone acetate.[78] In this study 83% of the subjects reported that their hair fall ceased after three months on the drug and 77% of the cases noticed hair regrowth.

Spironolactone is the drug often prescribed for women with polycystic ovarian syndrome (PCOS) due to its ability to block the DHT receptors in the hair follicle. PCOS causes the same hair loss that men have as it is also caused by an excess of androgens.

There are some contraceptive pills that contain CPA plus oestrogen which may be a better option for a woman showing early signs of FPHL than pills containing progesterone plus oestrogen.

There are many scientists who believe that androgens do not play any part in female hair loss. In one study there was no observed predictor of a positive response to spironolactone including patient age, menopause status, serum ferritin, serum hormone levels, clinical presentation or any other disease parameters.[79]

This would explain why some women find spironolactone helpful but the majority do not.

Finasteride (Propecia)

Propecia, also sold as Proscar, is a drug taken orally for the treatment of pattern baldness in men.

Propecia works by decreasing the concentration of dihydrotestosterone (DHT) in the blood and therefore the scalp.

An elevated level of DHT, known colloquially as 'bad testosterone', is associated with benign prostatic hyperplasia (enlarged prostate), prostate cancer and a reduction in healthy hair follicles.[80]

So, while it would seem to be an open and shut case, hormones are a delicate and tricky matter and there are not a lot of reliable and straightforward ways to medically influence them without causing other problems. For example, some men experience sexual side effects such as erectile dysfunction and decreased libido when taking finasteride.

In order to gain FDA approval for use in treating hair loss, controlled clinical studies must be carried out to prove efficacy and safety. Hence, several clinical studies have been performed on men using Propecia.[81] The results, while positive, are not overwhelming.

Low doses of finasteride taken over five years have been shown to reduce the concentration of DHT in the blood, having a positive effect on both preventing hair loss and triggering regrowth. However the degree of improvement is fairly minimal. Average regrowth was 2% and that was in men with mild to moderate hair loss.[82]

According to Section 14.2 of the FDA label for Propecia, a small study was also carried out on post-menopausal women. In this study 137 women were treated with Propecia or a placebo over a period of 12 months. At the end of the trial, they were unable to demonstrate any improvement in hair count as self reported by the participants – nor was it visible in submitted before and after photos.[83]

Finasteride isn't the baldness cure we would like to believe. You can find more information about the studies that were carried out in Section 14 of the FDA label on the FDA website.[84]

Importantly, Propecia in not approved by the American FDA for use by women because it is known to cause birth defects in the unborn male foetus. The drug's label warns that women who are pregnant or may become pregnant **must not handle** this drug under any circumstances.

Given that Propecia is not recommended for women, a study by Harvard Medical School in 2003 [85] found that consuming soy products and/or black tea did inhibit the production of DHT – perhaps more useful information for us that a benefit could come in the form of a daily cuppa with creamy soy milk.

Flutamide

Flutamide is a nonsteroidal anti-androgen that needs to be prescribed by a doctor. It is mainly used in the treatment of prostate cancer because of its testosterone (androgen) blocking action. Its main function for hair loss, therefore, is to block the androgen receptor. This treatment may be useful if a woman's hair loss is caused by an excess of DHT on the scalp but it won't be useful otherwise.

Combined treatments

All of the treatments mentioned here can and do make a difference for some women, under some circumstances. But their efficacy is limited if the underlying causes and/or triggers are still present, or if the therapy is not the correct treatment for the issue. This may account for the wide range of results noted in the studies conducted on these various treatment therapies.

There is an explosion of companies online offering tailor-made and over-the-counter hair loss pills to men and women following an online consultation with a 'licensed physician'.

While it would appear (according to the marketing) that many of these tailor-made (compounded) tablets that you can purchase following an online consultation may have some positive therapeutic effect, they could also be helping women via a placebo effect. Under the care of a doctor who understands hair loss and who prescribes a medication you believe is exactly right for you, and given the mental anguish associated with female hair loss, it would not be surprising that a psychosomatic benefit occurs throughout the process and prescription.

These compounded tablets generally contain minoxidil, spironolactone and some hair health vitamins and nutrients. We know that spironolactone can have some effect and minoxidil too will help many women in some way. We also know that some vitamins and nutrients do influence hair growth and loss but that they are likely to only be effective if there is an established deficiency. So, an individually prescribed pill is unlikely to contain anything more than the ingredients you can buy over the counter yourself or after consultation with your primary care physician.

While you can pay an online hair loss specialist a fee each month for a personal combination prescription, you could also arm yourself with a solid understanding of your underlying causes and the nutritional aspects associated with your hair loss and work on it yourself.

The internet is full to overflowing with both competent doctors and charlatans selling the dream of a full head of hair to women. These online sellers know that women will stop at almost nothing to get their hair back.

So, please do your research before relying on online hair loss doctors and their medications.

INVASIVE PROCEDURES

Platelet-rich plasma

One of the latest seeds of hope to arise from the scientific community is platelet-rich plasma (PRP) for female hair loss. It sounds very sci-fi and very promising in the marketing. Many women have jumped on the PRP bandwagon.

Here's the research on PRP – what it is and how it works.

What is PRP?

You may recall from biology classes that blood is made up of plasma, red blood cells, white blood cells and platelets. You may also remember that platelets are responsible for clotting the blood during illness or injury. But what you may not know is that plasma contains hundreds of proteins called growth factors, which are capable of stimulating cellular growth, proliferation, healing and cellular differentiation. Sounds promising for hair regrowth, doesn't it?

Patients who receive PRP treatment undergo two to three harvests, where blood is taken and the plasma is separated out from the other components. They are then re-injected with their own blood which has been 'improved' to contain a specific concentration of platelets – roughly five times the typical baseline level.

The theory behind PRP treatments is that adding platelets, and therefore growth factors, to the blood increases cellular activity; and the more cellular activity, the more hair will grow. Simple, right?

Well . . .

Does PRP regrow hair?

First, let's get one thing straight: nothing can regrow hair where there are no hair follicles to work with. That's a fact.

The only way you can have hair again in bald areas is to take active hair follicles from somewhere else on the body or scalp and transplant them there. This is why hair transplants are still widely used to increase the amount of hair on the head.

There have been a few scientific studies on the effectiveness of PRP treatments for hair regrowth but they have only utilised small sample sizes.

One small study carried out on 23 males found a mean increase in total hair density of 45.9 (number of hairs/cm^2) following three months of regular PRP treatments.[86]

Another randomised controlled trial published in 2020 divided both male and female participants into 2 groups. The participants were treated with PRP each month for 3 months. 3 months later at the follow up appointment, both groups showed an increase in hair density.[87]

Is PRP suitable for women?

There is no reason why PRP wouldn't be suitable for women but bear in mind that the current clinical research has been based on extremely small sample sizes and there were very few women involved in these studies.

A word of caution: PRP treatment increases the growth of all the cells it comes into contact with. This means, for example, that if there are any skin cancer cells in the vicinity, these too could also be influenced to grow faster. It is also worth noting that the earlier this therapy is applied the more likely it is to be successful.

What is the process?

PRP treatment first involves having blood taken, usually from the arm.

This blood is then put into a machine that separates out the platelets from the other blood cells via a process called centrifugation. These isolated platelets are then re-injected subcutaneously (just under the skin surface) back into the patient's scalp. Mesotherapy is usually the method used: a non-surgical treatment that can be carried out in a doctor's rooms. It consists of multiple tiny injections that are used to transfer the platelet-rich plasma into the area of the scalp where thicker hair is desired.

This process is repeated during three to four treatments over a five to six week period, with each treatment taking up to 90 minutes. If there are signs of good results then the treatment will need to be repeated every 3 to 6 months to continue producing a benefit. PRP treatments for hair loss must be ongoing to remain effective. Once the treatment stops the decline in hair thickness will continue where it left off.

Over time, the hair growth around the PRP-treated area may also become sparse and new areas may need treatment. Thus, once hair loss has advanced to a certain level, PRP treatments may produce an uneven aesthetic result.

Since the 1970s, PRP has been used in various clinical applications including cardiology, sports medicine, cosmetic surgery and pain management. It is only recently that it has begun to be used as a hair regrowth procedure. Over the past 5 years there has been a significant increase in the number of clinical studies carried out using PRP on participants with hair loss and it does certainly show some promising results

Hair plucking

A huge amount of buzz arose a few years ago, relating to a possible breakthrough in follicle regeneration. It centred around the somewhat counterintuitive idea that plucking hairs could actually result in more hair growth.

Should we all be grabbing the tweezers and intentionally balding ourselves in the pursuit of a full, thick head of hair?

The study

Scientists studied the regeneration of hair follicles in response to patterned hair plucking in mice. They discovered that by plucking 200 hairs in a specific pattern in a limited area, more than 1,000 hairs grew back in their place, as well as in nearby regions.[88] Interestingly, if the hairs were plucked from random spots or over larger areas, this level of regeneration did not occur.

Why did this happen?

The researchers concluded that the affected hair follicles were able to 'communicate' a kind of distress signal to surrounding follicles, signifying threat. These follicles then responded by regenerating as many as five times the amount of replacement hair.

This phenomenon is similar to the way that bacteria functions. Bacteria are able to communicate with each other through a chemical signalling system called quorum sensing. They use this to detect when their numbers are strong enough to achieve their objective.

Can plucking really help hair loss?

This finding was a big breakthrough for science but according to the lead researcher (Cheng-Ming Chuong M.D., Ph.D. of the Keck School of Medicine, Dept of Pathology, University of Southern California) more research is needed to determine whether these animal findings may translate to strategies for combating hair loss in humans.[89]

Although many hair loss bloggers cite this study as the 'breakthrough we have all been waiting for', it does seem to be a likely red herring. Still, here's hoping that these findings lead to further study that proves this technique really is the breakthrough we're all ready for.

Hair transplants

A hair transplant, also known as hair restoration surgery, is a procedure where hair is taken from an area on the head where there is healthy hair and then transplanted onto a thinning or balding area.

There are two different types of hair transplants. The first and most popular is the follicular unit transplant (FUT) which involves taking skin with the hairs attached and grafting that skin to the new area. The second and supposedly less scarring option is a follicular unit extraction (FUE) where the surgeon takes only the follicles themselves and using a punch hole, transplants the individual follicles to the new area.

The FUE does leave a scar, in fact it leaves many scars as each punch hole has the potential to scar. The FUT also leaves a scar which is usually very fine and covered by the new hair growth.

These procedures are very painstaking, can only be done by a qualified surgeon and take a long time, anything up to 8 hours is not unusual.

They are tried and tested procedures that have been perfected over many years and generally produce very good outcomes. Perhaps the only downside is the cost.

There are also new robotic restoration devices which can perform a procedure similar to the FUE, but with greater precision. It will be interesting to watch what happens in this space, because from what I've seen of other robotic surgeries, the outcomes are so much better and more predictable than the manual equivalent.

COSMETIC SOLUTIONS

Scalp micropigmentation

Scalp micropigmentation is a permanent cosmetic solution which is achieved with a tattoo applied to the skin on the scalp where there is hair thinning and visible scalp. This can be a fabulous solution for a woman where the scalp is showing through the hair. If the hair loss continues, then more tattoos would need to be applied.

Many men who are entirely or nearly completely bald, shave what hair they have left and have micropigmentation done to their entire scalp, so it looks like they have a full head of hair that they have elected to shave.

Hair fibres

One 'secret' to instantly thicker hair is in a shake! Hair fibre concealers are available in easy-to-apply packs and a sprinkle to your roots may be the cosmetic solution you've been looking for.

Hair fibres are tiny, hair-like microfibres that come in a variety of hair colours. They are applied to fine, thin and thinning hair at the roots to instantly make the hair appear thicker. The latest technology hair fibres are made from cotton.

How do you apply hair fibres?

Simply shake onto dry hair and lightly blend in with the fingertips to disperse the fibres down the hair shaft. Hair fibres can be applied to hair following your usual styling products. As long as your hair is dry the fibres will cling.

High quality hair fibres stay in place in wind and light rain until they are washed out with shampoo. Some women like to use a hair spray to keep their fibres in place but generally you will find that products like Boost N Blend don't require a fixing spray. Hair fibre products that do require a fixing spray are most likely using outdated keratin technology.

How to apply hair fibres to a widening part

A widening part is often the most noticeable hair loss issue for a woman and it is the easiest to camouflage.

First part your hair parallel and about half a centimetre (an eighth of an inch) away from your actual part line. Shake in the hair fibres onto that line and then repeat on the other side of your part. You may not need to add in any fibres to your part line at all as this technique will disperse fibres to the hair on either side of your part and will virtually make your part line disappear.

If you feel your part line it too obvious for this technique, a zig zag part line can often fix that.

How do they work?

Hair fibres are slightly electrostatic. This is how they cling to dry hair, surrounding the hair shaft itself to make it appear up to 10 times thicker. Boost N Blend employs cutting edge technology to create hair fibres made from cotton. These are considered the superior option because cotton is colourfast and non-irritating. In addition, cotton hair fibres have a far superior cling factor compared with keratin fibres. They are more readily electrostatic (think of pulling a jumper over your head), which creates an instant 'cling' factor.

Hair fibres using keratin are made from animal fur or hair, which require a lot of chemical and antibiotic treatments to make them suitable for human cosmetic use. These products are then claimed to mimic the type of keratin found in human hair.

But the problem with keratin technology is that the resulting chemical cocktail in their formulation is water soluble and known to dissolve in sweat. When it dissolves, it turns . . . green!

They can also be sticky and clump on the scalp, and are known to cause irritation and itchiness for many users.

Cotton hair fibres, on the other hand, are vegan, natural and derived from the cotton plant. Since we wear cotton next to our skin every day, we already know it is non-irritating.

Can cotton hair fibres be detected? Will anyone know?

Boost N Blend hair fibres look completely natural, by design. They blend in with natural hair so successfully that they are virtually undetectable.

Applied correctly and with careful shade selection they can't even be seen in close range.

Don't worry, your secret is safe.

Boost N Blend was designed by women, for women. We carefully selected our shades based on real women's hair colours. Men's hair fibres have been on the market for a long time but male hair is different to women's in both texture and shade. Cotton hair fibre products like Boost N Blend, designed and made specifically for women, provide the best result because they were formulated for women's hair textures and shades.

How do I know which colour to choose?

Always choose the colour closest to your root colour. If in doubt, or you can't decide between two colour choices, select the darker option. Darker roots are more flattering and effective on women with thinning hair.

What if my roots are grey?

In this case, choose the colour you dye your hair.

One great additional benefit of cotton hair fibres is that they cover up the grey root colour, and many ladies find they get another week or so between dyes.

Are hair fibres waterproof?

Hair fibres generally stay in place in wind and rain. But since they wash out when you wash your hair, they will not stay in if you go swimming. One great tip, to both help if you do go swimming and also if you have a large area to cover, is to use a root cover up product (like Rootz) to paint onto your scalp before you apply fibres. This has the dual benefit of helping to make the fibres look even thicker but importantly, Rootz is waterproof. So if your fibres come off then the Rootz will remain as a scalp cover should it be needed.

Are there any side effects?

No, unless you are allergic to cotton.

Boost N Blend hair fibres do contain some other ingredients to ensure that the fibres cling to the hair and also to colour them. But it is very rare for someone to experience any negative side effects or reactions.

Do hair fibres clog the follicles and prevent further hair growth?

There is a lot of misinformation on this topic online. I have been using cotton hair fibres for over 10 years and in that time I have grown my hair back several times. I have had a few bouts of TE and on each occasion, I continued to use Boost N Blend every day. As my hair thinned out, I needed to use more. And even with using more and still using it every day, my hair grew back.

I do recommend you check the ingredients in your hair products as I have previously mentioned, to ensure that there are no nasty ingredients to compromise your hair health.

Will cotton hair fibres work on completely bald spots?

Hair fibres are designed to cling to hair – even the finest, almost invisible hair.

To manage a completely bald spot the best option is to grow your hair to brush over it, then 'thicken up' the hair using hair fibres. This can visibly disguise the patch.

Why haven't I heard of hair fibres before?

Helping women with hair loss is my business, and I get asked this question often. The answer is simply that no-one had made a product like this for women, until I did! There are a lot of keratin-based products on the market, mainly designed for men. Many of these will feature women using the product on their website and marketing materials but the reality is these products were designed by men, for men.

In 2013, I got together with an Australian hair colour specialist and designed hair fibres for women myself – in women's hair colours and with women's hair texture in mind. This is what became the Boost N Blend range.

Is it easy to adjust to wearing hair fibres?

Cotton hair fibres stay in place no matter what you do – even while you sleep.

By way of a personal experience, I often experience high wind on the weekends when I am boating – one of my favourite pastimes. The first time this happened when I was wearing my fibres, I raced for the on-board toilet mirror to check my hair. I was delighted to find that even after half an hour of blustering high wind the fibres hadn't budged.

More recently during a flood emergency I was stranded in the pouring rain for a few hours. As soon as I was able to do so, I ran for the nearest mirror to check my fibres were still in place and indeed they were.

If you want to see what a huge difference cotton hair fibres make, head over to the Boost N Blend website at www.boostn-blend.com where you will see many 'before' and 'after' photos that will give you an idea of what you can expect after one application. They really do make an enormous difference.

GETTING ON WITH LIFE

Now, to getting on with life. I really find it heart breaking listening to and reading the stories of women for whom hair loss has caused a detrimental change in their way of life.

I know you may feel that your level of attractiveness is, or was, reliant on your hair. Or that attractiveness lies solely in your appearance. I understand. I used to feel the same way.

But I think we all know instinctively that beauty does come from within. A smile, a happy face and a loving, giving personality all go a long way.

And the truth is, the people who know you well and who love you, will love you no matter what you look like.

There is so much you can do aesthetically to camouflage hair loss – from toppers to wigs, to hair extensions, to hair fibres and brush-on concealers. Then there are hair styles that will help, and scarves, hats and accessories for not only covering hair loss but creating modern fashion looks.

All of these elements will help deeply with building self-confidence. I don't think people notice our thinning hair as much as we think they do, especially with only even a small amount of effort to restyle or camouflage. After living with hair loss now for over 15 years and noticing whether people look at my head or not, I can honestly say people do not notice, and I don't think they noticed when my hair loss was at its all-time worst either.

We do put a lot of pressure on ourselves to be perfect or to look how we used to look. To look younger or slimmer or to have the hair of our teenage years. But the reality is, ageing well is such a great look. Being healthy on the inside radiates through to our smile and to our skin.

It may take a long time, even years to get your hair back, if ever. So, take everything you have learned in this book, digest it all and begin or continue your hair health journey with knowledge.

But above all, be consistent. There is no quick fix, it takes time for your body to heal and then to concentrate again on growing hair.

And here's my final piece of advice and my all-time number one tip:

Be good looking.

Be *good* at *looking* at the people around you. Notice people, say hello, say thank you to someone who serves you or steps aside to let you pass. Notice the small things that people do for you and for others. Smile at someone who passes you, smile at someone you ordinarily may not think to smile at, smile at a complete stranger. Make their day.

And this always leads to the bonus kind of good looking. Smiling at people, thanking people, acknowledging people who do things for you, has a rebound effect. When someone smiles back at you, that smile reflects on your face. It's kind of like the good looking multiplier effect. Smiling at others, being spontaneously kind radiates outwardly from our faces and to be perfectly honest, that's the best kind of good looking there is.

It tells people so much more about who we are.

We are so much more than our hair or our perceived imperfections.

I do hope I've been able to help you understand your body and your hair better. I hope that after reading this book, you will have gained something you didn't have before. Whether it's a newfound love of breathing, or the desire to throw those expensive supplements in the bin and work on your health more naturally.

Or perhaps it's the ability to stop, rest, de-stress and be good looking. Whatever it is, I hope that your hair days ahead will be less bumpy.

Bambi

NOTES

1   Female Hair Loss Help https://femalehairlosshelp.com/

2   Bambi Staveley, How to Make Thin Hair Fat, Barrallier Books Pty Ltd, Victoria, Australia, 2016

3   Lawlor DA, Davey Smith G, Ebrahim S (June 2004). "Commentary: the hormone replacement-coronary heart disease conundrum: is this the death of observational epidemiology?". Int J Epidemiol. 33 (3): 464–467. doi:10.1093/ije/dyh124. PMID 15166201.

4   Raghvendra K. Dubey, Bruno Imthurn, Lefteris C. Zacharia, and Edwin K. Jackson, Hormone Replacement Therapy and Cardiovascular Disease, Hypertension. 2004;44:789–795

5   Scheinfeld, Noah, 'A review of hormonal therapy for female pattern (androgenic) alopecia', Dermatology Online Journal, 2008,

6   Hoover E, Alhajj M, Flores JL. Physiology, Hair. [Updated 2021 Jul 26]. In: StatPearls [Internet]. Treasure Island (FL): StatPearls Publishing; 2022 Jan-. Available from: https://www.ncbi.nlm.nih.gov/books/NBK499948/

7   Randall, V. A., & Ebling, F. J. G. (1991). Seasonal changes in human hair growth. *British Journal of Dermatology*, 124(2), 146–151. doi: 10.1111/j.1365-2133.1991.tb00423.x.

8   Trüeb RM, Rezende HD, Dias MFRG. A Comment on the Science of Hair Aging. Int J Trichology. 2018 Nov-Dec;10(6):245-254. doi: 10.4103/ijt.ijt_56_18. PMID: 30783331; PMCID: PMC6369639.

9   Redler S, Messenger AG, Betz RC. Genetics and other factors in the aetiology of female pattern hair loss. Exp Dermatol. 2017 Jun;26(6):510-517. doi: 10.1111/exd.13373. PMID: 28453904.

10   Hamilton, James. (2005). Male hormone stimulation is prerequisite and an incitant in common baldness. American Journal of Anatomy. 71. 451 - 480. 10.1002/aja.1000710306.

11   P M Ramos, H A Miot, 'Female pattern hair loss: a clinical and pathophysiological review', *Journal of the Brazilian Society of Dermatology*, 2015;90(4):529-543. doi:10.1590/abd1806-4841.20153370

12   S Orme, D Cullen, & A Messenger. (1999). 'Diffuse female hair loss: are androgens necessary?' *British Journal of Dermatology*, 141, 521–523, 1999 *doi. org/10.1046/j.1365-2133.1999.03049.x,*

13   R Sinclair, 'Diffuse hair loss', *Journal of Dermatology* 38: 8–18. doi. org/10.1046/j.1365-4362.1999.00003.x_1999

14   R Sinclair, 'Diffuse hair loss', *Journal of Dermatology* 38: 8–18.doi. org/10.1046/j.1365-4362.1999.00003.x_1999

15   Bhat YJ, Saqib NU, Latif I, Hassan I. Female Pattern Hair Loss-An Update. Indian Dermatol Online J. 2020 Jul 13;11(4):493-501. doi: 10.4103/idoj. IDOJ_334_19. PMID: 32832434; PMCID: PMC7413422.

16   Chumlea WC, Rhodes T, Girman CJ, Johnson-Levonas A, Lilly FR, Wu R, Guo SS. Family history and risk of hair loss. Dermatology. 2004;209(1):33-9. doi: 10.1159/000078584. PMID: 15237265.

17   Redler S, Messenger AG, Betz RC. Genetics and other factors in the aetiology of female pattern hair loss. Exp Dermatol. 2017 Jun;26(6):510-517. doi: 10.1111/exd.13373. PMID: 28453904.

18   Sharpley CF, McFarlane JR, Slominski A. Stress-linked cortisol concentrations in hair: what we know and what we need to know. Rev Neurosci. 2011 Dec 8;23(1):111-21. doi: 10.1515/RNS.2011.058. PMID: 22150070; PMCID: PMC3381079.

19   Jacob KD, Noren Hooten N, Trzeciak AR, Evans MK. Markers of oxidant stress that are clinically relevant in aging and age-related disease. Mech Ageing Dev. 2013 Mar;134(3-4):139-57. doi: 10.1016/j.mad.2013.02.008. Epub 2013 Feb 18. PMID: 23428415; PMCID: PMC3664937.

20   Halliwell B. The antioxidant paradox: less paradoxical now? Br J Clin Pharmacol. 2013 Mar;75(3):637-44. doi: 10.1111/j.1365-2125.2012.04272.x. PMID: 22420826; PMCID: PMC3575931.

21   Grymowicz M, Rudnicka E, Podfigurna A, Napierala P, Smolarczyk R, Smolarczyk K, Meczekalski B. Hormonal Effects on Hair Follicles. Int J Mol Sci. 2020 Jul 28;21(15):5342. doi: 10.3390/ijms21155342. PMID: 32731328; PMCID: PMC7432488.

22   Jason Fung, *The Obesity Code,* Greystone Books,Canada *2016*

23   Hadshiew IM, Foitzik K, Arck PC, Paus R. Burden of hair loss: stress and the underestimated psychosocial impact of telogen effluvium and androgenetic alopecia. J Invest Dermatol. 2004 Sep;123(3):455-7. doi: 10.1111/j.0022-202X.2004.23237.x. PMID: 15304082.

24   Chaolin Huang, MD, Lixue Huang MD, Yeming Wang, MD, Xia li, MD, Lili Ren, PhD, Xiaoying Gu, PhD et al, '6-month consequences of COVID-19 in patients discharged from hospital: a cohort study', *The Lancet* Vol 397, Issue 10270, 2021

25   Sharquie KE, Jabbar RI. COVID-19 infection is a major cause of acute telogen effluvium. Ir J Med Sci. 2021 Aug 31:1–5. doi: 10.1007/s11845-021-02754-5. Epub ahead of print. PMID: 34467470; PMCID: PMC8407603.

26   Chaolin Huang, MD, Lixue Huang MD, Yeming Wang, MD, Xia li, MD, Lili Ren, PhD, Xiaoying Gu, PhD et al, '6-month consequences of COVID-19 in patients discharged from hospital: a cohort study', *The Lancet* Vol 397, Issue 10270, 2021

27   Deloche C, Bastien P, Chadoutaud S, Galan P, Bertrais S, Hercberg S, de Lacharrière O. Low iron stores: a risk factor for excessive hair loss in non-menopausal women. Eur J Dermatol. 2007 Nov-Dec;17(6):507-12. doi: 10.1684/ejd.2007.0265. Epub 2007 Oct 19. PMID: 17951130.

28   Tosti A, Piraccini BM, Sisti A, Duque-Estrada B. Hair loss in women. Minerva Ginecol. 2009 Oct;61(5):445-52. PMID: 19749676.

29   Tosti A, Piraccini BM, Sisti A, Duque-Estrada B. Hair loss in women. Minerva Ginecol. 2009 Oct;61(5):445-52. PMID: 19749676.

30   Australian Bureau of Statistics 'Australian Health Survey: Biomedical Results for Nutrients', 2011-12

31   Patel DP, Swink SM, Castelo-Soccio L. A Review of the Use of Biotin for Hair Loss. Skin Appendage Disord. 2017 Aug;3(3):166-169. doi: 10.1159/000462981. Epub 2017 Apr 27. PMID: 28879195; PMCID: PMC5582478.

32   US Food and Drug Administration, Safety Communication Update 11 May 2019

33   US Food and Drug Administration, Information for Consumers on Using Dietary Supplements, Questions and Answers on Dietary Supplements updated 22 July, 2019.

34   Mishra S, Stierman B, Gahche JJ, Potischman N. Dietary supplement use among adults: United States, 2017–2018. NCHS Data Brief, no 399. Hyattsville, MD: National Center for Health Statistics. 2021. DOI: doi.org/10.15620/cdc:101131.

35 https://www.goldsteinresearch.com/report/global-beauty-supplements-market-outlook-2024-global-opportunity-and-demand-analysis-market-forecast-2016-2024

36 Ekelem C, Pham C, Atanaskova Mesinkovska N: A Systematic Review of the Outcome of Hair Transplantation in Primary Scarring Alopecia. Skin Appendage Disord 2019;5:65-71. doi: 10.1159/000492539

37 Trüeb, R. M. (2003). Association between smoking and hair loss: another opportunity for health education against smoking? *Dermatology* (Basel, Switzerland), 206(3), 189–191. doi: 10.1159/000068894.

38 Peters EMJ, Müller Y, Snaga W, et al. Hair and stress: A pilot study of hair and cytokine balance alteration in healthy young women under major exam stress. *PLoS One.* 2017;12(4):e0175904. Published 2017 Apr 19. doi:10.1371/journal.pone.0175904

39 Department of Dermatology, University Hospital Hamburg-Eppendorf, University of Hamburg, Martinistrasse 52, 20246 Hamburg, Germany *Burden of hair loss: stress and the underestimated psychosocial impact of telogen effluvium and androgenetic alopecia*

40 unilad.co.uk/health/neuroscientist-reveals-how-to-access-your-brains-reset-button Accessed May 2022

41 Ma X, Yue ZQ, Gong ZQ, Zhang H, Duan NY, Shi YT, Wei GX, Li YF. The Effect of Diaphragmatic Breathing on Attention, Negative Affect and Stress in Healthy Adults. Front Psychol. 2017 Jun 6;8:874. doi: 10.3389/fpsyg.2017.00874. PMID: 28626434; PMCID: PMC5455070.

42 bbc.co.uk/programmes/articles/1mW6885X3N2gKnVjXT00KCj/how-to-reset-your-brain-with-your-breathing

43 Grant JE, Chamberlain SR. Trichotillomania. Am J Psychiatry. 2016 Sep 1;173(9):868-74. doi: 10.1176/appi.ajp.2016.15111432. PMID: 27581696; PMCID: PMC5328413.

44 Søsted H, Agner T, Andersen KE, Menné T. 55 cases of allergic reactions to hair dye: a descriptive, consumer complaint-based study. Contact Dermatitis. 2002 Nov;47(5):299-303. doi: 10.1034/j.1600-0536.2002.470508.x. PMID: 12534535.

45 Oliver, D. (2015). Why You Should Be Cautious Of Taking Biotin For Your Hair, Skin & Nails, The Huffington Post. Retrieved from http://www.huffingtonpost.com/2013/09/30/biotin-hair-skin-nails_n_4016804.html Accessed 28 April 2015

46 Patel DP, Swink SM, Castelo-Soccio L. A Review of the Use of Biotin for Hair Loss. Skin Appendage Disord. 2017 Aug;3(3):166-169. doi:

10.1159/000462981. Epub 2017 Apr 27. PMID: 28879195; PMCID: PMC5582478.

47   Cho YH, Lee SY, Jeong DW, Choi EJ, Kim YJ, Lee JG, Yi YH, Cha HS. Effect of pumpkin seed oil on hair growth in men with androgenetic alopecia: a randomized, double-blind, placebo-controlled trial. Evid Based Complement Alternat Med. 2014;2014:549721. doi: 10.1155/2014/549721. Epub 2014 Apr 23. PMID: 24864154; PMCID: PMC4017725.

48   Hajhashemi V, Rajabi P, Mardani M. Beneficial effects of pumpkin seed oil as a topical hair growth promoting agent in a mice model. Avicenna J Phytomed. 2019 Nov-Dec;9(6):499-504. doi: 10.22038/AJP.2019.13463. PMID: 31763209; PMCID: PMC6823528.

49   Scheinfeld, Noah, 'A review of hormonal therapy for female pattern (androgenic) alopecia', Dermatology Online Journal, 2008,

50   Almohanna HM, Ahmed AA, Tsatalis JP, Tosti A. The Role of Vitamins and Minerals in Hair Loss: A Review. Dermatol Ther (Heidelb). 2019 Mar;9(1):51-70. doi: 10.1007/s13555-018-0278-6. Epub 2018 Dec 13. PMID: 30547302; PMCID: PMC6380979.

51   Almohanna HM, Ahmed AA, Tsatalis JP, Tosti A. Review. Dermatol Ther (Heidelb). 2019 Mar;9(1):51-70. doi: 10.1007/s13555-018-0278-6. Epub 2018 Dec 13. PMID: 30547302; PMCID: PMC6380979.

52   MacFarquhar JK, Broussard DL, Melstrom P, Hutchinson R, Wolkin A, Martin C, Burk RF, Dunn JR, Green AL, Hammond R, Schaffner W, Jones TF. Acute selenium toxicity associated with a dietary supplement. Arch Intern Med. 2010 Feb 8;170(3):256-61. doi: 10.1001/archinternmed.2009.495. PMID: 20142570; PMCID: PMC3225252.

53   Banihashemi M, Nahidi Y, Meibodi NT, Jarahi L, Dolatkhah M. Serum Vitamin D3 Level in Patients with Female Pattern Hair Loss. Int J Trichology. 2016 Jul-Sep;8(3):116-20. doi: 10.4103/0974-7753.188965. PMID: 27625563; PMCID: PMC5007917.

54   Nowak K, Ratajczak-Wrona W, Górska M, Jabłońska E. Parabens and their effects on the endocrine system. Mol Cell Endocrinol. 2018 Oct 15;474:238-251. doi: 10.1016/j.mce.2018.03.014. Epub 2018 Mar 27. PMID: 29596967.

55   chemicalsafetyfacts.org/dmdm-hydantoin-2/ Accessed 5 May 2022

56   de Groot AC, van Joost T, Bos JD, van der Meeren HL, Weyland JW. Patch test reactivity to DMDM hydantoin. Relationship to formaldehyde allergy. Contact Dermatitis. 1988 Apr;18(4):197-201. doi: 10.1111/j.1600-0536.1988. tb02802.x. PMID: 3378426.

57   US Food and Drug Administration, www.fda.gov/cosmetics/cosmetic-ingredients/allergens-cosmetics#common. Accessed May 2022

58   Campaign for Safe Cosmetics www.safecosmetics.org/get-the-facts/chemicals-of-concern/ethanolamine-compounds/ Accessed May 2022

59   Campaign for Safe Cosmetics, www.safecosmetics.org/get-the-facts/chemicals-of-concern/petrolatum/

60   Author, 'article title', *International Journal of Trichology*, issue, year Gavazzoni Dias MF, de Almeida AM, Cecato PM, Adriano AR, Pichler J. The Shampoo pH can Affect the Hair: Myth or Reality? Int J Trichology. 2014 Jul;6(3):95-9. doi: 10.4103/0974-7753.139078. PMID: 25210332; PMCID: PMC4158629.

61   Monselise A, Cohen DE, Wanser R, Shapiro J. What ages hair? Int J Womens Dermatol. 2015 Oct 9;1(4):161-166. doi: 10.1016/j.ijwd.2015.07.004. PMID: 28491982; PMCID: PMC5419772.

62   Oh JY, Park MA, Kim YC. Peppermint Oil Promotes Hair Growth without Toxic Signs. Toxicol Res. 2014 Dec;30(4):297-304. doi: 10.5487/TR.2014.30.4.297. PMID: 25584150; PMCID: PMC4289931.

63   Murata K, Noguchi K, Kondo M, Onishi M, Watanabe N, Okamura K, Matsuda H. Promotion of hair growth by Rosmarinus officinalis leaf extract. Phytother Res. 2013 Feb;27(2):212-7. doi: 10.1002/ptr.4712. Epub 2012 Apr 20. PMID: 22517595.

64   T. W. Fischer MD,U. C. Hipler PhD,P. Elsner MD, Effect of caffeine and testosterone on the proliferation of human hair follicles in vitro, International Journal of Dermatology, January 2007 https://doi.org/10.1111/j.1365-4632.2007.03119.x

65   Prager N, Bickett K, French N, Marcovici G. A randomized, double-blind, placebo-controlled trial to determine the effectiveness of botanically derived inhibitors of 5-alpha-reductase in the treatment of androgenetic alopecia. J Altern Complement Med. 2002 Apr;8(2):143-52. doi: 10.1089/acm.2002.8.143. Erratum in: J Altern Complement Med. 2006 Mar;12(2):199. PMID: 12006122.

66   Pekmezci E, Dundar C, Turkoglu M. Proprietary Herbal Extract Downregulates the Gene Expression of IL-1 in HaCaT Cells: Possible Implications Against Nonscarring Alopecia. Med Arch. 2018 Apr;72(2):136-140. doi: 10.5455/medarh.2018.72.136-140. PMID: 30302033; PMCID: PMC6126931.

67   www.fda.gov/cosmetics/cosmetic-products/hair-smoothing-products-release-formaldehyde-when-heated

68   www.ph.news.yahoo.com/dry-shampoo-bad-hair-two-185509290.html

69   www.theatlantic.com/health/archive/2016/07/
the-unfortunate-reality-of-dry-shampoo/489989/

70   Suchonwanit P, Thammarucha S, Leerunyakul K. Minoxidil and its use in
hair disorders: a review. Drug Des Devel Ther. 2019 Aug 9;13:2777-2786.
doi: 10.2147/DDDT.S214907. Erratum in: Drug Des Devel Ther. 2020 Feb
10;14:575. PMID: 31496654; PMCID: PMC6691938

71   Dr Russell Knudson, The Hair Loss Show. YouTube https://youtu.be/
jztEaZKVziY

72   Dr Russell Knudson, The Hair Loss Show. YouTube https://youtu.be/
jztEaZKVziY

73   Avci P, Gupta GK, Clark J, Wikonkal N, Hamblin MR. Low-level laser
(light) therapy (LLLT) for treatment of hair loss. Lasers Surg Med. 2014
Feb;46(2):144-51. doi: 10.1002/lsm.22170. Epub 2013 Aug 23. PMID:
23970445; PMCID: PMC3944668.

74   Kim, Hyojin MD[1, 2]; Choi, Jee Woong MD[1]; Kim, Jun Young MD[3]; Shin,
Jung Won MD[1]; Lee, Seok-jong MD, PhD[3]; Huh, Chang-Hun MD,
PhD[1,*] Low-Level Light Therapy for Androgenetic Alopecia: A 24-Week,
Randomized, Double-Blind, Sham Device–Controlled Multicenter Trial,
Dermatologic Surgery: August 2013 - Volume 39 - Issue 8 - p 1177-1183 doi:
10.1111/dsu.12200

75   Pinar Avci, MD, Gaurav K. Gupta, MD, PhD, Jason Clark, MD, Norbert
Wikonkal, MD, PhD,and Michael R. Hamblin, PhD. Low-level laser (light)
therapy (LLLT) for treatment of hair loss. Lasers in Surgery and Medicine
9999:1 (2013)

76   Dr Russell Knudson, The Hair Loss Show. YouTube https://youtu.be/
g6vIjxHUHOY

77   Sinclair R, Wewerinke M, Jolley D.Treatment of female pattern hair loss
with oral antiandrogens. Br J Dermatol. 2005 Mar;152(3):466-73. PubMed
Scheinfeld,

78   Coneac A, Muresan A, Orasan MS. Antiandrogenic Therapy with
Ciproterone Acetate in Female Patients Who Suffer from Both
Androgenetic Alopecia and Acne Vulgaris. Clujul Med. 2014;87(4):226-34.
doi: 10.15386/cjmed-386. Epub 2014 Nov 12. PMID: 26528029; PMCID:
PMC4620668.

79   https://escholarship.org/uc/item/3b81s01s Scheinfeld, N. (2008). A review
of hormonal therapy for female pattern (androgenic) alopecia. Dermatology

Online Journal, 14(3). http://dx.doi.org/10.5070/D33b81s01s Retrieved from https://escholarship.org/uc/item/3b81s01s

80 Kinter KJ, Anekar AA. Biochemistry, Dihydrotestosterone. [Updated 2022 Mar 9]. In: StatPearls [Internet]. Treasure Island (FL): StatPearls Publishing; 2022 Jan-. Available from: https://www.ncbi.nlm.nih.gov/books/NBK557634/

81 US Food and Drug Administration https://www.accessdata.fda.gov/drugsatfda_docs/label/2012/020788s020s021s023lbl.pdf accessed May 2022

82 Jonathan Darrow, Finasteride as an FDA-Approved Baldness Remedy: Is It Effective? https://blog.petrieflom.law.harvard.edu/2013/01/31/finasteride-as-an-fda-approved-baldness-remedy-is-it-effective/

83 US Food and Drug Administration https://www.accessdata.fda.gov/drugsatfda_docs/label/2012/020788s020s021s023lbl.pdf accessed May 2022

84 US Food and Drug Administration https://www.accessdata.fda.gov/drugsatfda_docs/label/2012/020788s020s021s023lbl.pdf accessed May 2022

85 Zhou JR, Yu L, Zhong Y, Blackburn GL. Soy phytochemicals and tea bioactive components synergistically inhibit androgen-sensitive human prostate tumors in mice. J Nutr. 2003 Feb;133(2):516-21. doi: 10.1093/jn/133.2.516. PMID: 12566493; PMCID: PMC2683253.

86 Gentile P, Garcovich S, Bielli A, Scioli MG, Orlandi A, Cervelli V. The Effect of Platelet-Rich Plasma in Hair Regrowth: A Randomized Placebo-Controlled Trial. Stem Cells Transl Med. 2015 Nov;4(11):1317-23. doi: 10.5966/sctm.2015-0107. Epub 2015 Sep 23. PMID: 26400925; PMCID: PMC4622412.

87 Shapiro J, Ho A, Sukhdeo K, Yin L, Lo Sicco K. Evaluation of platelet-rich plasma as a treatment for androgenetic alopecia: A randomized controlled trial. J Am Acad Dermatol. 2020 Nov;83(5):1298-1303. doi: 10.1016/j.jaad.2020.07.006. Epub 2020 Jul 9. PMID: 32653577.

88 Chen CC, Wang L, Plikus MV, Jiang TX, Murray PJ, Ramos R, Guerrero-Juarez CF, Hughes MW, Lee OK, Shi S, Widelitz RB, Lander AD, Chuong CM. Organ-level quorum sensing directs regeneration in hair stem cell populations. Cell. 2015 Apr 9;161(2):277-90. doi: 10.1016/j.cell.2015.02.016. PMID: 25860610; PMCID: PMC4393553.

89 Chen CC, Wang L, Plikus MV, Jiang TX, Murray PJ, Ramos R, Guerrero-Juarez CF, Hughes MW, Lee OK, Shi S, Widelitz RB, Lander AD, Chuong CM. Organ-level quorum sensing directs regeneration in hair stem cell populations. Cell. 2015 Apr 9;161(2):277-90. doi: 10.1016/j.cell.2015.02.016. PMID: 25860610; PMCID: PMC4393553.

Printed in Australia
AUHW020834051022
369807AU00003B/3

9 781922 890245